100
THINGS YOU
CAN DO TO STAY
FIT AND HEALTHY

100
THINGS YOU
CAN DO TO STAY
FIT AND HEALTHY

Simple Steps to Better Your Body and Improve Your Mind

Scott Douglas

Skyhorse Publishing

Skyhorse Publishing books may be purchased in bulk at special discounts for sales promotion, corporate gifts, fund-raising, or educational purposes. Special editions can also be created to specifications. For details, contact the Special Sales Department, Skyhorse Publishing, 307 West 36th Street, 11th Floor, New York, NY 10018 or info@skyhorsepublishing.com.

Skyhorse® and Skyhorse Publishing® are registered trademarks of Skyhorse Publishing, Inc.®, a Delaware corporation.

Visit our website at www.skyhorsepublishing.com.

10 9 8 7 6 5 4 3 2 1

Library of Congress Cataloging-in-Publication Data is available on file.

Cover design by Tom Lau
Cover photo image: iStockphoto

Unless otherwise indicated, all images: iStockphoto

Print ISBN: 978-1-5107-1235-5
Ebook ISBN: 978-1-5107-1236-2

Printed in China

Table of Contents

Foreword

There is no shortage of health advice. We are deluged daily with products and programs that profess to have the "secret" formula. Reading too much or study alone leaves us with analysis paralysis. In my twenty-eight years of work with people's health issues, I've witnessed amazing results once a person is ready to step into the driver's seat of their own health process.

Not all of us possess the genetics to be in the triple-digit age club, or even aspire to live that long, but we all share a basic need to enjoy good health that enriches the quality of our lives. We now know we can change our brain and body chemistry through aerobic exercise, strength training, meditation, healthy nutrition, and countless other strategies. Research is rife with documentation of the healing benefits of these simple strategies that bring well-being.

Outsourcing a healthy lifestyle process is costly and ultimately unsustainable. Once you take the leap to embrace simple, small incremental changes, and then integrate these strategies into your lifestyle, true transformative results are harvested.

Scott Douglas—a man who values his own health journey enough to spend a considerable amount of his busy work day incorporating these doctrines—truly lives his beliefs. Scott begins each day practicing these simple self-care principles: running, restoring, aligning, fueling, and rejuvenating his body to invest in his health.

A true health advocate, Scott has been engaged in a lifelong pursuit of optimum health and fitness. I've had the privilege to run the roads, sample the fresh local food, and witness his impeccable journalistic integrity and relentless research stamina. I'm certain you'll find the 100 tips in this book to be both enjoyable and beneficial. Enjoy them in good health.

—Phil Wharton,
President of Wharton Health Solutions

Introduction

The best time to plant a tree was twenty years ago. The second best time is now.

This Chinese proverb says a lot about improving health. Ideally, you established good habits decades ago. If you did, you're more likely to be healthy and happy today. But if you didn't, then right now is the best time to make some changes. And even if you already do a lot of the right things, like being active, eating well, and managing stress, there are things you can start doing immediately to be even healthier. After all, nobody has ever wished they were less healthy.

This book is focused on simple steps you can take today to improve your health and fitness. In many cases, you'll see almost immediate benefits. This is not to imply that I'm providing one-and-done easy fixes. Good health is a lifelong goal, and therefore a lifelong undertaking. Rather, the ideas in this book are manageable, realistic practices that, when you make them a regular part of your life, will help you feel better today and be in even better health years from now. Think of them as you would small but consistent investments into a retirement account. At any one time, what you're doing might not seem dramatic or important. But over time, as your good habits build on one another, you'll have a growing fund of wealth or, in this case, health.

I've divided the hundred tips in this book into five chapters, each focused on an aspect of your health: general, cardiovascular, muscular/skeletal, internal, and mental. As you'll see, much of the advice will have benefits beyond its chapter's topic. To take just one example, finding an aerobic activity you enjoy doing (item #28) has obvious cardiovascular benefits. But regular aerobic exercise will also strengthen your muscles (and in some cases bones), reduce your risk of some cancers, and improve your mood.

Each of the 100 tips in this book is meant to be self-contained. Feel free to start reading from wherever you like, based on the areas of health you most want to improve. If you read front to back, however, you might notice a key theme emerging, as I did the more I prepared to write. You'll see several places where what's being recommended is a deliberate step away from the trappings of modernity. In the twenty-first century, we have a way of life that would be the envy of nearly every human who has ever lived. And yet we'll see several instances of our default mode of existence presenting a threat to our health. We're among the first people in human history who need to make an effort to move enough and not eat too much.

The recommendations in this book are based on combining authoritative health research with real-world concerns. If you want the latest fads or "secrets," this book might not be for you. If you want a distillation of reputable research into practical advice applicable to most people, keep reading.

A quick personal note: please don't think I see myself as a paragon of health doling out sermons from on high. I have more room for improvement than most people in two key areas, posture (item #46) and time spent sitting (item #4). Because of earlier neglect of flossing (item #25), I now have periodontal disease. When I get busy I have to remind myself I'll get more done and my mind will be calmer if I slow down and concentrate on one thing at a time rather multitask (item #85). And if it's ever discovered that eating peanut butter by the spoonful out of the jar causes cancer, I'm a goner.

Like you, I want to live my full allotment of years and feel vibrant while doing so. Consider me a fellow striver who, through personal curiosity and professional experience, has done the advance work for you on key ways to meet our mutual goal of a long, healthy life.

While you read this book and think about how to improve your health, heed the words of tennis legend Arthur Ashe: Start where you are. Use what you have. Do what you can.

CHAPTER 1

27 Things to Do to Improve Your General Health and Fitness

In this first chapter, we'll start with tips that have a global effect on your health or don't pertain to one of your body's internal systems.

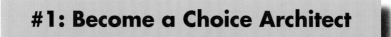

#1: Become a Choice Architect

Let's start with something that, in itself, won't improve your health, but will make it much more likely that you'll successfully enact some of the other 99 tips in this book.

Behavioral economists talk about the importance of choice architecture, or the environment in which we make choices. The classic example is the difference between an employer-matched retirement fund where participation requires choosing to enroll, versus enrollment as the default option. In the latter case, more employees participate. The gist of the field's teaching is to make it easy to do the right thing.

Choice architecture is key for daily and long-term success in healthy living. Knowledge is power, and I hope that this book will give you several ideas on simple steps you can take to almost immediately improve your health. But whatever you read here or elsewhere will remain more of an interesting factoid than life-changing guidance without the right environment in which to implement it.

Here's a personal example: one of my favorite tips in this book is #59, about strengthening the front neck muscles to be able to hold better head posture. I learned this simple exercise from four-time Olympian Meb Keflezighi, who recommends it as a way to improve running form. I've found it immensely helpful in relieving, and even preventing, the shoulder and upper-back pain I get when I spend too much time in front of my computer.

As I'm writing this sentence, a small green ball I use for the exercise is inches away on the table where I am working. Keeping the ball in sight and in reach reminds me to take a short break two or three times a day to strengthen my neck. If I kept the ball anywhere else, I'd be much less likely to do this exercise, no matter how good my intentions are.

Similar examples abound: Keep your pantry stocked with healthful staples so that when you're tired and famished, your default dinner isn't to have a pizza delivered. (See #75.) Keep a water bottle at your desk to make it more likely that you'll stay hydrated throughout the work day. (See #68.) Schedule exercise time as you do other appointments to increase the likelihood of it happening.

Surround yourself with people with similar health goals so that your preferred way of living seems normal. And so on. Set up your life so that it's easy to do the right thing for your health.

#2: Make More Than One Good Change at a Time

As I wrote in the introduction, this book is focused on small, simple steps you can take today to improve your health.

Simple isn't necessarily easy, however, especially when it comes to establishing new health habits. Change is always difficult. Yet as counterintuitive as it might seem, you'll probably make more progress by adopting a few new practices simultaneously than one step at a time.

Consider research from the University of California, Santa Barbara. In the study, half of the subjects transformed their lifestyles significantly, all at once: they worked out daily, kept a food journal to monitor their eating habits, and took time for stress-reduction mental exercises. The other half went about their standard collegiate ways. At the end of the study period, the several-things-at-once group were, of course, healthier and happier than the control group. What was surprising was that their increase in self-esteem and their performance on cognitive-function tests increased more than would have been expected if they had made just one big change, such as improving their diets.

The findings suggest that a few good new habits mixed together can create a positive-positive feedback cycle. Success in one area can motivate you in other areas, and success on one day can make it easier to do the right thing the following day.

Of course, you don't want to overwhelm yourself with lifestyle changes. Too much too soon can lead to abandoning the whole project. A solution for tackling a few changes at a time? When time permits and doing so makes sense, cluster good habits. In my sport, running, it's common for people to finish a run and do some stretching or strengthening while they're flushed with the feeling of a good workout. Then, while they're still in heightened self-care mode, they're more likely to have a good post-run meal and try to extend their currently calm mindset to the rest of the day's challenges. Along the same lines, you could easily integrate self-massage (#55), flossing (#25), and a screen-free bedroom (#6) into a healthful pre-sleep routine.

Inertia can be a difficult force to overcome, but once you've done so, it doesn't take much effort to keep your momentum going.

#3: Enjoy Your Morning Coffee

Coffee fans, rejoice! Unless you regularly drink more than five cups, your daily routine has many health benefits. Here's a brief overview.

Coffee's immediate effect on your mental state is well known and well-loved. (See #91 for more on that.) There appear to be long-term effects, as well. Research has found coffee drinkers to be at lower risk for depression and suicide. Coffee might also slow cognitive decline and the onset of Alzheimer's disease in later years.

According to the World Health Organization, coffee lowers your risk for liver and uterine cancer. Moderate intake has also been associated with a lower risk for heart disease, other types of liver disease, type 2 diabetes, Parkinson's disease, and even tinnitus.

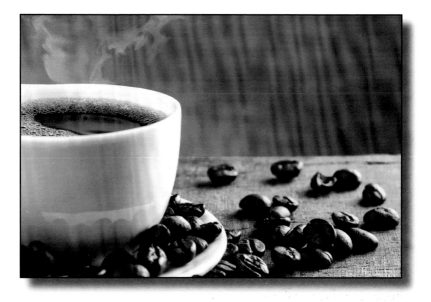

Large, long-term studies have also found that coffee drinkers are less likely to die than coffee abstainers during a given period.

This item on the health benefits of coffee could be much longer. But you don't really need me to convince you to drink some. And isn't it time for another cup?

#4: Sit Less

The health perils of being sedentary have been known for decades. What's come into sharper focus are the particular risks of a key part of the sedentary lifestyle. Sitting, we're increasingly learning, is really bad for you, even if you exercise regularly. The topic is such an area of concern that health researchers have coined the phrase "inactivity physiology" for the study of this hallmark of modern life.

Think about your typical day. You might drive to work, work at a desk for several hours, drive home, watch television, and pore over your phone. During those activities, and while eating, you're probably sitting. One estimate has the average American sitting thirteen hours a day. Assuming eight hours in bed, this means spending more than 80 percent of your waking hours sitting.

In Chapter 3, we'll see how too much sitting can harm your posture and even change how you walk. The focus of most research on sitting is how it can be an independent risk factor for many chronic diseases, such as diabetes, heart disease, and high blood pressure. That is, even when you account for other known risk factors, such as smoking, being overweight, or not exercising, the amount of time you sit can by itself make you more likely to have one of these conditions. To cite one of many examples: a study of more than 82,000 men grouped subjects by how much time outside work they watched television, sat at a computer, or read. Those who spent five or more hours per day in those sedentary activities were 34 percent more likely to have heart failure in an eight-year period than those who spent two or fewer hours per day in those ways.

That being the case, it's not surprising that excessive sitting has also been found to increase your risk for the worst condition of all—dying. Obviously, we're all going to die. When health researchers say that something increases your mortality risk, they mean within a given time period. In the case of sitting, one large-scale study of people in fifty-four countries estimated that sitting more than three hours a day contributed to more than 400,000 deaths in a nine-year period.

It's thought that excess sitting suppresses lipoprotein lipase, a substance in skeletal muscle that breaks down potentially harmful triglycerides. When lipoprotein lipase is unable to do its job as well, triglyceride and blood glucose levels can rise, and HDL cholesterol ("good" cholesterol) levels can fall. Those undesirable occurrences then increase your risk for the common conditions listed above.

One of the most interesting findings about sitting concerns what have come to be called "active couch potatoes," or people who exercise most days but otherwise spend most of their waking time sitting. It turns out that such people aren't immune to the risks of excess sitting. One study looked at the sitting habits of almost 1,000 men who all had a high level of cardiorespiratory fitness (i.e., the type improved by aerobic activities such as jogging, cycling, hiking, and swimming). Even though the men were similarly fit and active, those who spent the most time sitting were 1.65 times as likely during the ten-year study period to develop metabolic syndrome (diabetes, high blood pressure, cardiovascular disease, etc.). The bottom line: If you exercise regularly, keep at it. If you don't, start. But either way, don't think your workouts cancel out the bad effects of sitting.

There aren't yet official guidelines on how much sitting is too much. There is, however, widespread agreement that most of us do too much of it. You certainly aren't going to harm your health by sitting less. When in doubt, get out of your chair. Doing so at least once an hour is thought to lessen lipoprotein lipase suppression. Moving about for a few minutes—walking across the room, doing stretching exercises, squats, push-ups, etc.—is best. If that's not possible, at least stand and move in place. At home, stand at least part of the time while doing things like being on the phone, watching television, and reading.

#5: Get Enough Sleep

People seem to enjoy telling others how little they sleep. The tales often have an undertone that equates not sleeping much with being more productive. The facts about sleep deprivation say otherwise, at least if you care about the quality of what you're doing during all that time awake.

In the short term, sleep deprivation leads to impaired cognitive function, memory, and alertness, even after just one night of inadequate sleep. It's been shown to double the risk for on-the-job injuries and is estimated to contribute to at least 100,000 car crashes and more than 1,500 fatalities a year. More subjectively, sleep deprivation leads to being more impulsive, irritable, indecisive, clumsy, and hungry.

Long-term sleep deprivation has serious health consequences, including an increased risk for high blood pressure, stroke, heart disease, immune system compromise, obesity, and depression. It's also been linked with a greater risk of dying in a set time period than people who sleep more.

There's no universal necessary amount of sleep, which makes it easier for people to convince themselves they're getting enough. That said, most adults do best with between seven and nine hours of sleep per day. In the research mentioned above about increased mortality risk with long-term sleep deprivation, those who were at greater risk of dying in a given period reported getting fewer than six or seven hours per day.

One sign that you're sleep-deprived is, paradoxical though it might sound, that you fall asleep almost instantly. This includes when you enter a dark environment such as a movie theater during daylight hours. Other signs include relying on an alarm clock to wake, feeling sleepy when driving, relying on caffeine to get through your days, difficulty focusing with your eyes, and not feeling rested when you get out of bed.

Sometimes, periods of sleep deprivation are inevitable. Research suggests that if you know you have such a period coming up, such as a crunch time at work or a days-long conference, you can bank sleep and lessen the effects of later reduced sleep. In one study, people who slept extra in the six days before going without sleep for twenty-four hours performed better on a physical test than they did when they followed their normal sleep patterns for the six days preceding an all-nighter. Another interesting takeaway from the study is how the participants got extra sleep—they went to bed two hours earlier than usual. Doing so didn't lead to tossing and turning until they normally fell asleep. On average, the participants slept an additional seventy-five minutes a night when they went to bed early.

#6: Make Your Bedroom a Screen-Free Zone

Do you take your phone into the bedroom at night? If so, you're part of a strong majority—depending on what survey you read, somewhere between two-thirds and three-quarters of American adults say they go to bed with their phone within reach, with the proportion even greater in people under the age of thirty.

While this practice is great for keeping up with what's going on with your friends and social media, it's not good for your sleep patterns, and by extension your health.

For starters, there's the just-one-more-text phenomenon that can mean staying up later than you otherwise would. Even if you're cooing over pet photos rather than getting riled up by someone's political posts, your brain is engaged and stimulated. Think about how much easier it is to fall asleep when you're calm and relaxed versus dealing with a racing mind.

More specific to phones, tablets, laptops, and the like, the blue light that these gadgets emit is at a wavelength that interferes with your body's secretion of melatonin, a hormone that helps to regulate your circadian rhythms. Exposure to blue light in the evening has been shown to delay the release of melatonin, with the result that your body thinks it's not yet time to fall asleep. Then, once you

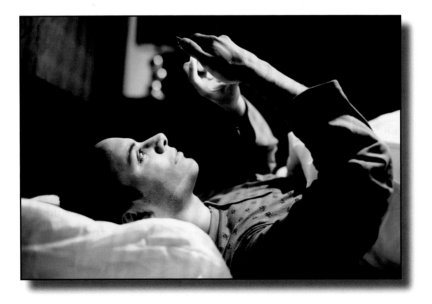

do fall asleep, your body secretes melatonin later than it otherwise would, and you can wake feeling groggy.

Try keeping phones and other devices with screens out of your bedroom and see if your sleep improves. If you don't notice a difference after a week or two, take the next step and institute a curfew—no gadget use in the hour before you plan to go to bed.

#7: If You Need to Lose Weight, Start with a Small Goal

A full plan on losing excess weight is outside the scope of this book. What I can offer is the heartening fact that even small losses can have big health benefits.

A study at Washington University looked at what happened when obese people lost 5 percent of their weight. That figure is lower than what's often prescribed as necessary to make beneficial changes kick in.

After losing 5 percent of their weight, the subjects' insulin sensitivity, blood pressure, heart rate, and triglyceride levels improved significantly. Those improvements lowered the subjects' risk of complications from type 2 diabetes and cardiovascular problems.

Of course, this doesn't mean that if you have significant weight to lose you should shed 5 percent and stop trying. In the study, as in many others, as the subjects went to losses of 10 percent and greater, their health continued to improve, not just in the measures above, but also in things like markers of inflammation. The more the subjects lost, the more there were simultaneous improvements in several internal organs.

Still, setting incremental goals is always better than an all-or-nothing approach. After all, you didn't reach your current weight overnight. Take pride in each accomplishment, and let your progress motivate you to more success.

#8: Eat a Good Breakfast

Here are a few reasons breakfast has earned its reputation for importance. (Notice I didn't say "most important." Meals are like your children—love them all equally.)

After any meal, your blood sugar rises, and then your pancreas produces insulin to move the sugar into your cells for them to use as energy. Having steady blood sugar means that your levels are relatively flat throughout the day (there will also be some increase after eating), in which case your energy level shouldn't fluctuate greatly during the day.

When you wake, you've probably gone without calories for longer than any other stretch in a twenty-four-hour period. If you then don't eat until midday, your blood sugar level will continue to fall throughout the morning. Then when you do have lunch, your blood sugar level will rise much more rapidly than if you'd eaten breakfast. Over time, having large variations in blood sugar levels reduces your insulin sensitivity—glucose doesn't enter your cells as easily, so it builds up in your blood. Reduced insulin sensitivity can lead to developing type 2 diabetes.

In contrast, research has found that people who regularly eat breakfast have improved insulin sensitivity, with the result that their blood sugar is more stable after all meals.

Many other benefits have been linked to having more stable blood sugar levels, including being more active before noon and having improved cognitive functioning on tasks like memory, attention, and processing speed in the morning. Most studies have found that breakfast eaters have better-quality diets than breakfast skippers. Some studies have found that breakfast skippers wind up eating more total calories in a day than breakfast eaters.

If you're not a breakfast eater and have no appetite in the morning, bear in mind that breakfast doesn't have to be large. A small bowl of cereal or yogurt and fruit might contain 500 to 600 calories, or about a quarter of most people's daily needs. Like all meals, a good breakfast supplies a balance of protein, carbohydrates, and fat.

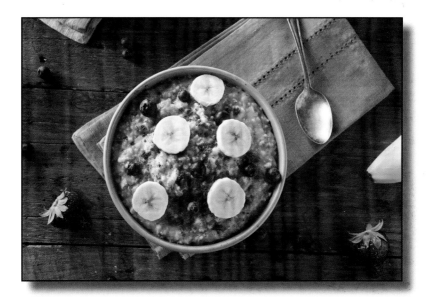

#9: Breathe from Your Belly

You'll keep on breathing as long as you live without ever having to think about it, but that doesn't necessarily mean that you're breathing in the best way. Nor does it mean that you can't permanently alter your breathing pattern.

Breathing is an example of what's known as an autonomic process, or one that your nervous system performs without conscious effort. That's in contrast to something like walking across the room, which is a voluntary process that you decide to undertake. Other examples of autonomic processes are heart rate and digestion.

Most of us do what is called apical breathing, in which your chest is the primary mover. See for yourself: take a breath and notice where most of the action is. If you're like most people, to inhale you pulled your chest and lungs up, as if you were drawing up air from your throat with a straw. When you exhaled, your upper chest moved back down and your stomach was more pushed out than when you inhaled.

Contrast that with how a baby naturally breathes. If you happen to have one handy, you'll see her stomach inflate with each breath in, then return to its normal position during exhalation. This is belly breathing. It makes much better use of the diaphragm, the large, flat muscle just below the lungs that helps to draw air into the lungs. When you belly breathe, the diaphragm contracts properly, moving down, thereby making more room for your lungs to fill with air.

The cells in your body need oxygen to function properly and are harmed by carbon dioxide. So drawing in more oxygen and expelling more carbon dioxide with each breath can have a profound effect on your health. Everything from digestion and posture to work capacity and even your mental state improves when you belly breathe.

Switching to belly breathing will take conscious effort at first. You can hasten the process by practicing in bed before you go to sleep. While lying on your back, place one or both hands on your stomach, near your belly button. Inhale by gently expanding your belly, from both the front and sides. Watch to see how your hands rise as you breathe in, then fall as you exhale. Do some breaths through your mouth and nose, and others only through your nose, to better learn how to use this technique at all times.

Once you're familiar with what belly breathing should feel like it, practice it throughout the day. If you're doing something that doesn't require much concentration, check in on your breathing. Commit to belly breathe for the next little while. Another good time to practice is when you feel stressed. If you're stuck in traffic, or on hold with the cable company, or just got an upsetting text, take deep belly breaths, and notice how focusing on really filling your lungs with air and then exhaling completely helps to calm you. With regular practice, belly breathing will become your natural method.

#10: If You Smoke, Stop Today

Everyone knows that smoking is one of the worst things you can do for your health. It leads to heart disease, strokes, high blood pressure, emphysema, at least sixteen types of cancer, and a host of other diseases and conditions. Cigarettes have been described as the only product that, when used as directed, are designed to kill you.

What's not universally agreed upon is how best to kick the habit—gradually reduce the number of cigarettes you smoke, or stop all at once? Recent research suggests going cold turkey gives you a greater chance of success.

In a study published in 2016, almost 700 adults considered to be addicted to tobacco underwent one of two forms of smoking-cessation treatment. Half of them gradually reduced their smoking by 75 percent over a two-week period before quitting. The other half stopped all at once. Both groups received behavioral support and used nicotine gum.

One month after the day they quit, 39 percent of the gradual-reduction group were succeeding in not smoking. In comparison, 49 percent of those who quit immediately were still abstaining one month later.

Six months after quitting, some members of both groups had resumed smoking. But the ones who stopped immediately were still

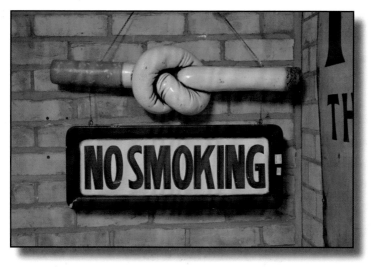

Image Via Creative Commons.

more successful (22 percent remained abstinent) than the gradual reducers (15 percent remained abstinent).

Whichever route you choose, try to line up professional and personal support, and consider a product such as nicotine gum. Good luck.

#11: Don't Chew Tobacco

Chewing tobacco is often considered not as unhealthful as smoking tobacco. That might be technically true, but in a practical sense only in the way that three whacks in the head with a wrench isn't as bad as five. There is simply no safe level of tobacco use.

The health risks of chewing tobacco are many. For starters, it's possible to absorb more nicotine from chewing tobacco than smoking. That increases the chances that you'll get addicted to nicotine, and either face a difficult struggle to break the addiction or suffer one or more of the many consequences of chewing.

As is the case with smoking, those consequences include a greater risk for some types of cancer. For chewing tobacco, the most common types are esophageal and oral, with the latter including cancer of the mouth, tongue, cheek, throat, and gums. Chewing tobacco has also been linked to an increased incidence of pancreatic cancer. The spots in your mouth where you place chewing tobacco are at greater risk of developing a type of lesion that can turn cancerous.

Even if you don't develop cancer, chewing tobacco wreaks havoc on your mouth. The sugar in chewing tobacco can lead to more cavities. You're also more susceptible to gum disease, especially in the areas where you put the tobacco, and subsequent tooth decay and tooth loss.

#12: And While We're At It, Don't Vape

Electronic cigarettes haven't yet been proven to be as disastrous for your health as traditional forms of smoking and chewing tobacco. That's primarily because they entered the market unregulated, and little is known about what substances specific products contain. Manufacturers must now register with the Food and Drug Administration but have until 2018 to submit an application detailing their products' contents.

The executive summary of what is known is that electronic cigarettes impart no health benefits, while subjecting users and bystanders to harmful chemicals and putting users at risk for nicotine addiction.

Electronic cigarettes contain a battery, heating element, and cartridge. Inside the cartridge is nicotine that's been extracted from tobacco and mixed with a base, liquids, and flavorings. After the cartridge is lit, users inhale the burned substances and then exhale a vapor (hence the term "vaping").

One of the two main concerns with vaping is the nicotine, a highly addictive substance. Studies have found the amount of nicotine in electronic cigarettes to vary widely. The amount of nicotine delivered also differs among devices. Nicotine has been shown to

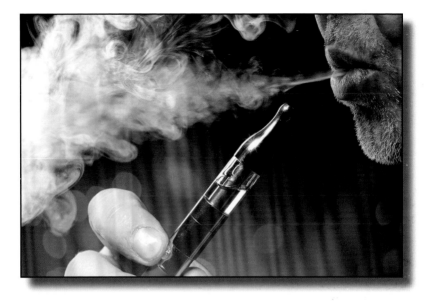

hurt maternal and fetal health, and impair brain development in children and adolescents. It can also cause cardiovascular problems.

The big unknown about electronic cigarettes is what chemicals are in the cartridge liquid. What has been learned isn't good. The FDA has found known carcinogens and toxins in products it has tested. Some of the flavoring chemicals are known to be harmful when consumed. Other flavoring chemicals are safe when added to foods but have not been shown to be safe when inhaled through electronic cigarettes.

Analyses of the emissions of electronic cigarettes have found formaldehyde and other known carcinogens and toxins, strongly suggesting that exposure to others' vaping is dangerous.

Health experts say that conventional, proven tobacco-cessation programs are preferable to vaping for people who are trying to quit traditional smoking.

#13: Have Indoor Plants

You might be surprised to hear that, as part of its mission to understand the outer reaches of the universe, NASA has been a leader in quantifying the health benefits of indoor plants.

In 1973, NASA launched Skylab, the first US space station. Also that year, NASA discovered that the synthetic materials used to construct Skylab were off-gassing, or emitting low levels of chemicals. In all, NASA identified more than 100 volatile organic chemical compounds, or VOCs, in the air inside Skylab. With known irritants and carcinogens among the chemicals found in Skylab's air, the situation was unacceptable, given that the space station was by necessity a closed environment.

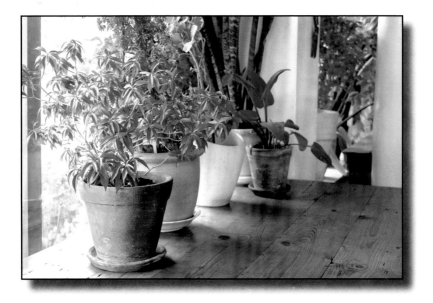

Part of the solution? Plants. NASA found that several types of plants, led by various palms, largely removed the VOCs from the air and improved the overall air quality within Skylab.

This phenomenon has been observed in more common environments. What's called "sick building syndrome" occurs when occupants of a building report symptoms such as skin rashes, irritated eyes, allergic reactions, and fatigue only during the time they're in a particular building. It's believed that a less extreme, but still significant, version of the Skylab situation underlies sick building syndrome—low-level off-gassing of harmful chemicals in a poorly ventilated space.

That being the case, it stands to reason that plants can work their air-purifying magic just as well in your hermetically sealed office as in outer space. Indoor plants can also absorb sound and thereby lower noise levels, a welcome benefit in most open-plan offices. If you get resistance from your higher-ups, have them google studies that have found increases in productivity of as much as 15 percent when plants are added to an office.

At home, you probably have more control over your space's ventilation. There's still good reason to have indoor plants there, especially in the winter. Indoor greenery has been shown to act as a natural humidifier, counteracting the dry air that can afflict your skin and breathing during the months when you're most likely to keep windows and doors closed.

On the basis of NASA's research, experts advise fifteen to eighteen plants in a 1,800-square feet living space, or two plants per 100 square feet in a building with normal-size (up to 10 feet) ceilings.

Of more than fifty plants that have been tested, the following are among those that rate highest for removing airborne chemicals:

palms, ficus, florist's mum, gerbera daisy, English ivy, tulips, dend-robium orchard, and spider plants.

Talking to plants might help them. Having indoor plants to talk to will definitely help you.

#14: Avoid Pesticides on Produce

There's a compelling reason for buying organic produce on the basis of nutritional quality. But even if there weren't, many people would opt for organics because of the chemicals sprayed on produce when it's grown conventionally, especially by large-scale farms that supply mass-market grocers.

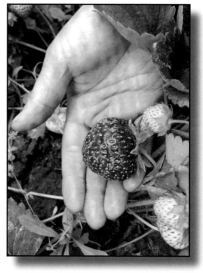

Consider: According to the US Department of Agriculture, more than 80 percent of conven-tionally grown produce is sprayed with a class of insecticides called organophosphates. While these pesticides are effective at limiting crop damage by insects, they don't distinguish between pests and humans. Exposure has been linked to dizziness, nausea, other short-term symptoms, and, because levels can build in the body over time, more long-term issues such as cancer and nerve damage. And that's from just one common class of pesticide.

If this is a concern—and it probably should be!—then the obvious thing to do is avoid buying produce that's been sprayed with harmful pesticides. That, however, isn't an economically viable choice for many people. In that case, you need to prioritize your purchases, which is where the Environmental Working Group's Dirty Dozen guide comes in handy.

It lists the twelve popular conventionally grown fruits and vegetables that, as commonly sold, are highest in pesticide residue. For the most recent testing period, they are strawberries, apples, nectarines, peaches, celery, grapes, cherries, spinach, tomatoes, sweet bell peppers, cherry tomatoes, and cucumbers.

As you can see, these are mostly items with relatively large edible surface areas that can easily absorb the pesticides. In contrast, the top three items on EWG's Clean Fifteen list, indicating low amounts of pesticide residue, are avocados, sweet corn, and pineapples. All have a barrier between the plant's exterior and the part you eat.

The EWG produces wallet-size versions of its lists that are convenient to consult when you're shopping.

The caution about large-scale pesticide use generally doesn't apply to produce grown conventionally on small farms, the sort you might buy from at your local farmers' market. An organic farmer once told me he'd rather buy produce from a small conventional farm than a large, mass-market organic operation. His reasoning was that the small conventional farms have relatively little land to work with. As such, they need to have a diversity of crops, so that if one crop fails, they have others to sell. This diversity lowers the need to aggressively go after one or two pests with large-scale spraying. In addition, the farmer told me, because small farms have relatively little land to work with, they need to treat it all lovingly. They're less likely to use pesticides that might help with this year's crops but that will damage the soil for future years.

If you're buying one of the items from the EWG's Dirty Dozen from a conventional farmer, ask about the farm's pest-treatment practices.

#15: Don't Microwave Food in Plastic Containers

Many people now avoid water bottles that contain bisphenoal A, an industrial chemical used to make some plastics and resins, and better known as BPA. The concern with BPA is that it can leak into the foods and beverages from the packaging containing those items. This is undesirable because exposure to BPA has been linked to some cancers, sexual dysfunction, brain damage, and other conditions.

Unfortunately, many of those same people unknowingly do something that increases their exposure to BPA when they pop leftovers in the microwave.

The National Institute of Environmental Health Sciences, which is part of the National Institutes of Health, advises against microwaving food in containers containing polycarbonate plastics, the type commonly found in the tubs and containers you might have in your cupboards for storing leftovers. Some frozen dinners are also packaged in containers with BPA.

Heating food in such containers, these experts say, increases the risk of BPA being released into your food as the plastics break down over time.

For the same reason, they recommend washing these containers by hand rather than in the dishwasher.

In independent tests, some plastics marketed as BPA-free have nonetheless been found to contain traces of the chemical. Given the uncertainty, this is a case where better safe than sorry is a reasonable plan of action while waiting for more information. That's especially so considering how easy it is to act differently to avoid the potential risk—store food in the non-plastic alternatives that are now available, put food to be reheated on a plate or in a bowl before microwaving, and keep plastics out of the dishwasher.

And let's face it, there are plenty of compelling reasons to skip frozen dinners already. Avoiding the potentially harmful packaging it can come in is another.

#16: Wear a Seat Belt

I won't insult your intelligence by telling you to avoid drinking and driving. I will risk doing so by reminding you of the importance of always wearing a seat belt. There aren't many simpler things you can do to preserve your health.

According to the National Safety Council, about 100 people die and 1,000 are seriously injured every day in the United States because of car crashes. In more than half of those deaths, the person won't be wearing a seat belt. Drivers under the age of twenty-five have the highest crash rates yet are also the least likely to wear seat belts. As a result, motor vehicle crashes are the leading cause of death among teens.

Seat belts protect you in two ways. First, in the initial few seconds after a crash, an unbelted person will continue to travel at the speed the vehicle was going at the time of impact. Imagine hurling your head at the dashboard at thirty miles per hour, or fifty, or seventy. Second, in addition to keeping you from colliding with a car part or other person, seat belts help you absorb the impact forces in the safest way possible. One study estimated that proper seat belt use (shoulder harness and waist belt) reduces the risk of death in a crash by 86 percent. Another calculated that proper seat belt use can almost cut in half the number of serious injuries.

Seat belt use is much less common in back seats, but just as important.

#17: Don't Drive Distracted

And while we're on the subject of driving…

As a society, we've made huge progress the last few decades in getting people not to drink and drive. Let's hope it doesn't take that long to get widespread buy-in on not driving distracted.

There are three forms of distracted driving—visual, manual, and cognitive. Talking and texting on your phone while driving can involve all three. (Because of the different attentional cues, your brain experiences a phone call differently than an in-person conversation.) Texting tends to lead to longer periods of distraction than talking on a phone or eating.

According to the Centers for Disease Control and Prevention, 424,000 people were injured in automobile crashes involving a distracted driver in 2013, almost 10 percent more than just two years earlier. The CDC attributes more than 3,000 fatalities a year to distracted driving. (The equivalent figure for drunk driving is a little less than 10,000.) Young drivers are especially prone to distracted driving. An American Automobile Association study found that almost 60 percent of teen crashes involved distracted driving.

Despite these statistics, many of us find ways to excuse our incidents of distracted driving—"It's just a short text," "I need to take this call," etc. There's almost always a way to justify "just this once." We see others texting and driving and shake our heads, but ignore that we look the same to others.

Yet when you consider that a car traveling at fifty-five miles per hour will cover the length of a football field in the time it takes to read an average text, "just this once" is enough to contribute to the stats. Other dangers of phone use while driving include dramatically slowed reaction times and drifting into other lanes. You also

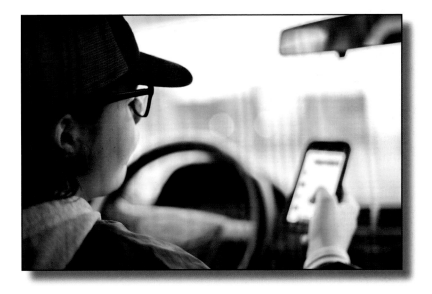

increase the chance of others hitting you—people tend to slow when texting and driving, thereby affecting the flow of traffic without other drivers having a way to know things are about to change.

Distracted driving is an instance where "just say no" is the universally right approach. Eat your meals and put on your make-up at home. If you absolutely must tend to a text or call while in the car, pull over first.

18: Protect Your Eyes from Computer and Other Screens

According to one Norwegian study on computer users, just two hours working on a laptop computer is enough to significantly increase these symptoms: eye-related pain and tiredness, blurred vision, itchiness, gritty eyes, light sensitivity, dry eyes, and tearing eyes. Think about that in light of recent estimates that the average person spends more than eight hours a day looking at computer, phone, and tablet screens.

The best cure is prevention; eye strain aside, most of us would benefit from less time bent over our phones. Your time in front of a computer screen might be much less under your control, in which case you need to mitigate exposure.

Lighting is key. First, if possible, make your computer the brightest source of lighting in the room. Reduce overhead lighting in favor of floor lamps. Try to have your screen to the side of rather than directly in front or back of windows. If you don't have much control of the lighting situation where you work, adjust the brightness setting on your computer so that it's similar to the ambient lighting. Keeping the screen clean helps to reduce glare.

Positioning is also important. The screen should be flat and directly in front of you, at about the length of a straight arm.

Like other body parts, eyes have muscles. Any muscle becomes tired and strained with overly repetitive use. At least every twenty minutes, take a twenty-second break and look at an object twenty feet away. While you're working, try to remember to blink frequently and normally to lessen dry eyes.

Finally, have an eye exam. Some of the fatigue your eyes feel from screen use might be because you need glasses or a different prescription.

#19: Watch Your Earbud Volume

If you've recently used a gas-powered lawnmower, eaten in a restaurant where you had to raise your voice to speak with your companions, or walked down a Manhattan street, think about how loud that situation was. The volume level of all three is typically about eighty-five decibels, generally considered the threshold for something that can be dangerous to your hearing.

Unfortunately, eighty-five decibels is also a common volume level for people listening to music or other audio content through earbuds. And unlike a biweekly mowing or occasional restaurant meal, wearing earbuds is for some people a daily occurrence.

Noise-induced hearing loss occurs when hair cells in the inner ear, which convert vibrations into electrical signals that the brain recognizes as sound, are damaged. This can occur either from a one-time event of extraordinary volume, such as a large gun or bunch of firecrackers going off close to your head, or through regular exposure to lower levels of still-too-loud sound.

The latter scenario is where earbuds can enter the picture. Wearing them while walking around town, riding public transportation, shopping, and working out can easily total an hour or more a day at potentially dangerous volume levels. That's especially so if you wear them in part to drown out environmental noise, such as when you want to hear your exercise playlist in a loud gym, in which case you probably turn up the volume more.

For earbud use, audiologists recommend keeping the volume level on your phone or other device at 60 percent or less most of the time. For most people this will mean being able to hear some environmental sound. Brief bouts (less than an hour at a time) louder

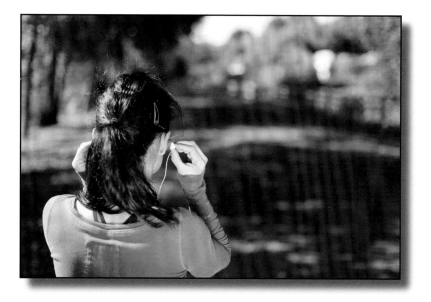

than that are okay, but of course not ideal. If one reason you tend to use a higher volume setting is to better hear the nuances of music—sound quality is compromised when audio files are converted to the standard MP3 format—consider investing in higher-quality earbuds. They will allow you to hear distinct tones at lower volumes.

#20: Don't Put Cotton Swabs in Your Ear Canal

It can be satisfying—in a gross kind of way—to dig around inside your ear and produce a wad of wax at the end of a cotton swab (the most famous brand of which is Q-tips). Don't do it. Extracting wax from your ear canal with a cotton swab solves no health problems while potentially creating some.

Earwax, technically known as cerumen, plays an important part in your ear's health. It helps to keep dust and other small particles from entering your eardrums. It's also thought to have an antibacterial role. Attempting to remove earwax is misguided, and using a cotton swab to do so can be counterproductive, because it can push earwax farther into the ear canal.

More significant, poking around within your ear can lead to infection and hearing loss.

There are times when earwax build-up and/or hardening, known as impaction, needs to be addressed. But cotton swabs are not the tools to use in this situation. Even the makers of Q-tips, who have a vested interest in widespread use of their product, don't encourage cotton swabs for this purpose. The Q-tips site touts the product's usefulness for "arts & crafts, manicures, makeup application, cleaning and more," with the cleaning elsewhere specified as hard-to-reach places in your home, not your inner ear. Cotton swabs can be safely used to gently clean the outer ear.

The symptoms of earwax impaction aren't unique to that condition. They include hearing loss, pain, dizziness, ringing in the ears, and a feeling of fullness in the ears. Over-the-counter softening ear drops can help to treat earwax build-up at home. If the above symptoms persist, especially pain and hearing loss, medical attention is warranted.

#21: Wear Sunscreen Year-Round

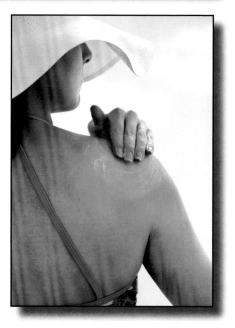

We all know that greater exposure to the sun's ultraviolet rays increases our risk of skin cancer. So I'll be brief here and convey a few facts about proper sunscreen use.

The sun emits ultraviolet rays year-round. On cloudy days, as much as 80 percent of ultraviolet rays reach your skin. Bottom line: wear sunscreen on exposed skin regardless of weather conditions or time of year.

Research has found that most people apply about 25 percent of the recommended amount of sunscreen. Picture a one-ounce shot glass. That's the amount to apply over the skin that will be exposed.

Notice the future tense of the previous sentence. Apply sunscreen fifteen minutes before going outside to allow for full absorption.

Use a sunscreen labeled as "broad spectrum," which means it protects against ultraviolet A and ultraviolet B rays. The American Academy of Dermatology recommends a sunscreen with an SPF of 30 or higher. The organization also advocates using a water-resistant sunscreen.

Sunscreens with high SPFs don't eliminate the need for proper use. A sunscreen with an SPF of 100 isn't three times more effective than one with an SPF of 30. Regardless of its SPF, sunscreen should be applied after two hours of outdoor time and/or situations such as swimming or heavy sweating that cause it to run off your skin.

If the risk of skin cancer isn't enough to induce sunscreen use, maybe vanity is. An Australian study looked at how sunscreen use affected skin aging among residents of Queensland, known as the Sunshine Coast. The researchers found that adults ages twenty-five to fifty who followed guidelines for sunscreen use had 24 percent less skin aging due to the sun (wrinkles and sagging skin) than adults of the same age who applied sunscreen as they saw fit.

Here are two additional sun-related thoughts. First, as we'll see in Chapter 4, some sunlight exposure is necessary to meet your vitamin D needs. Current evidence suggests that regular sunscreen users still absorb enough ultraviolet B rays to create sufficient vitamin D. Second, life is a balancing act—don't let fear of skin cancer prevent you from going outside, especially if that means you'll be less active.

#22: Keep Your Hands Clean

Having clean hands is one of the simplest, most effective ways to avoid getting sick (and making others sick).

In the past few years, hand-sanitizer dispensers have popped up everywhere. That's a good trend, but it shouldn't be taken to mean that hand sanitizer supersedes washing your hands with soap and water. The Centers for Disease Control and Prevention says that, in most cases, washing with soap and water is the best way to remove harmful microbes from your hands. Wash for at least 20 seconds under running water, rubbing vigorously to create friction.

Where hand sanitizer comes in, well, handy is when washing with soap and water isn't feasible. In those situations, proper use of the right type of hand sanitizer kills most types of germs, bacteria, and fungi. There are some key exceptions. According to the CDC, one germ against which hand washing is superior is norovirus, which most often causes vomiting and diarrhea in the winter. Washing your hands after using the bathroom and changing a diaper, and before cooking and eating, is key to slowing the spread of norovirus. Hand sanitizers are ineffective at removing the spores created by the *C. difficile* bacteria, which can cause conditions ranging from diarrhea to potentially fatal inflammation of the colon.

Hand sanitizers aren't as effective if they're not thoroughly applied in sufficient quantity. Accumulate a dime-size amount in the palm of one hand, and then rub over both sides of both hands, and between fingers, for thirty seconds. Effectiveness is also limited if your hands are dirty, because the soil or grime can be a barrier between the sanitizer and your skin.

It's also important to use the right type of hand sanitizer. The CDC says that hand sanitizers should contain between 60 percent and 95 percent alcohol.

Using hand sanitizer in combination with regular washing with water and soap appears to be especially effective. In one study, office workers who used hand sanitizer at least five times a day in addition to washing their hands were two-thirds less likely to get sick than their coworkers who only washed with soap and water.

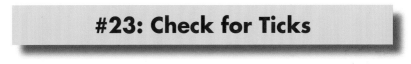

#23: Check for Ticks

Lyme disease is a mostly preventable infectious disease that, despite years of public education, remains highly prevalent. The Centers for Disease Control and Prevention estimates that more than 300,000

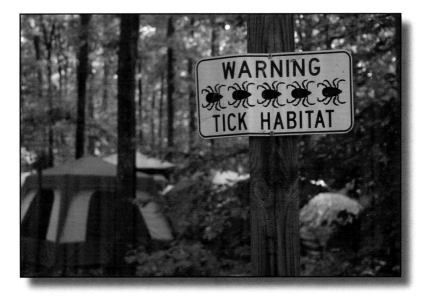

cases of the disease occur annually in the United States. Lyme disease is known for producing symptoms days or even months after its onset, with symptoms ranging from rashes and fatigue early on to arthritis and neurological problems, and even heart damage, later. Even after treatment, symptoms can linger for months.

Clearly, this is a disease worth avoiding. The best way to do so is to guard against and then diligently check for the blacklegged ticks whose bite transmits the disease. The ticks are most active between April and September but can be encountered at any time during the year.

Although many people consider Lyme disease a New England and Mid-Atlantic phenomenon, cases have been documented in all fifty states and the District of Columbia. So regardless of where you live, you'll want to take precautions when in the ticks' most common environments, woody areas with high grass and leaf litter. Before heading into the woods, apply an insect repellant that contains 20 to 30 percent DEET. While in the woods, stick to the center of the trail, where there's less opportunity for ticks to attach themselves.

Once you're out of the woods, check for ticks. Lyme disease is most often transmitted by nymphs, an immature stage when the tick is approximately one-quarter inch wide. So look carefully. Perform a full-body scan, either in front of a mirror or with the help of a companion. Look especially in areas with warm folds of skin, such as your armpits, ears, and backs of the knees, as well as your head and other hairy areas. Also check the clothing you had on, or better yet, wash it. Then shower to help remove any ticks that are loose.

If you have a dog, regularly check him for ticks. This is both for the dog's sake—dogs are highly susceptible to tick bites and tick-borne diseases—and yours. Many dogs like to veer off trails into exactly the type of areas where ticks are most prevalent. Ticks can then either attach themselves to the dog or remain loose and move to bedding or clothing before biting you.

#24: Wait to Brush Your Teeth After Eating

Wait, what? Aren't you being a paragon of virtue when you head right from the table to the sink and brush your teeth?

Alas, no. Here's why: the normal pH level in your mouth is 7, which is considered to be a neutral medium between acid and base. But when you eat, the pH level in your mouth becomes more acidic as bacteria on the enamel of your teeth metabolize food. This occurs especially after you've consumed acidic food or drink, such as alcoholic beverages, soda, fruit and fruit juice, and vinegar.

Brushing your teeth when your mouth is in this more acidic state doesn't help to return it to neutral. Instead, it can increase the potential destructiveness of the acids by pushing them farther into the enamel and the dentin, the layer below the enamel. The process is analogous to rubbing vigorously to get a wood stain to penetrate the pores of the wood.

The better approach is to wait about half an hour after eating before brushing. In that time, your saliva works to return the pH level of your mouth to neutral. To remove food from and between teeth soon after eating, floss. To hasten the return to a neutral pH level, rinse your mouth with water or an antibacterial mouthwash.

#25: Floss

You've been hounded your whole life about flossing, and now it's happening again. According to the American Dental Association, only 50 percent of Americans floss daily, and 18 percent do not floss at all. But it's important far beyond how your teeth will look your next time in the dentist's chair.

Flossing removes the bacterial build-up on and between your teeth. When that bacteria remains in your mouth, it can harden, at which point it's known as tartar. It can also lodge under your gums, and that's when the real trouble starts. What starts as gingivitis (inflamed gums) can progress to periodontal disease, in which the bacteria start to erode bone tissue in teeth. Unchecked periodontal disease is the leading cause of tooth loss in adults.

There's more: probably because of the chronic inflammation it subjects the body to, gum disease has been linked to higher-than-average rates of heart disease, stroke, and giving birth to low-weight babies. Clearly there's more benefit to flossing than removing that sesame seed from your morning bagel that has lodged between your front teeth.

The benefits of flossing are immediate, and the consequences of not flossing occur almost as quickly. In a study involving twins, one child from each set flossed daily, and the other didn't floss for two weeks. Their dietary and other health habits were similar. After just two weeks, the twins who didn't floss showed early signs of bacterial infection, while the twins who flossed didn't.

Given all that, it's hard not to justify devoting a minute or two a day to flossing.

#26: Plant a Garden

Gardening is a great reminder that meeting activity guidelines doesn't have to mean putting on workout gear and heading to the gym. During the growing season, labor-intensive gardening can go a long way toward totaling the 150 minutes per week of moderate activity the Centers for Disease Control and Prevention recommends.

Gardening will have you squatting and lifting, digging and toting, working your upper and lower body. Bonus: you'll be doing that outside and toward a tangible project that will yield visual and perhaps savory dividends.

As with so many worthwhile activities, gardening's physical benefits go hand in hand with mental ones. Gardening can bring

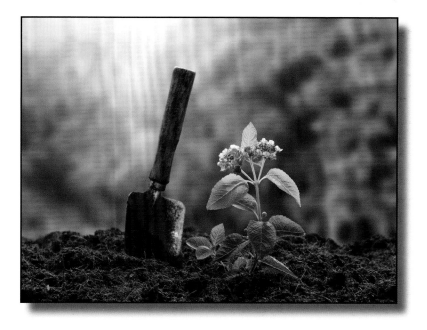

a state of focus and calm similar to what some people achieve via meditation. One study found that subjects experienced more stress relief from gardening than reading. (These gardeners must not have had many pests on their plants.) Gardening nicely satisfies the human urge to set and achieve goals.

You should, of course, plant whatever type of garden you want. But here's a vote in favor of growing vegetables, because of the nutritional value and unmatchable taste of peak produce picked just before you eat it.

#27: Redouble Your Health Practices in Times of Stress

When you hit a rough period—work overload, bad family news, etc.—it's easy to let your healthy lifestyle slip. All your focus is on getting through the crisis; good self-care feels like an indulgence you have neither the time nor mental energy for.

But these are exactly the times when your body most needs your attention. Light exercise, healthful meals, sound sleep, and quiet mental breaks will help to lower the levels of stress hormones coursing through your system. You'll wake better able to tend to your responsibilities than if you make self-defeating, self-fulfilling choices from the perspective that everything is going to hell, so what does it matter what you do?

During these periods, imagine that you're an athlete prepping for an important competition. Consider how your choices will later effect you. Instead of seeking comfort in junk food, eat healthful meals to bolster your body. Instead of blowing off your normal exercise routine, do at least an abbreviated version to reenergize yourself. Instead of drinking alcohol to forget your problems, have liquids that will keep you better hydrated and, therefore, more alert and able to deal with the current situation.

Other tips: resist the urge to go overboard on caffeine, lest you wind up that much more wired and tired. Take a few minutes a few times a day, including before going to bed, to sit quietly and calm your mind. Find something diverting to read before bed to help you fall asleep. (Ideally, your reading material will be print, not digital, so that you can sleep better. See item #6.)

Committing to good health practices during times of stress has an important psychological component. Taking care of yourself in these situations is a way of telling yourself that, as bad as things are, you're maintaining some control over your life. That mindset, in turn, can help you better assess the situation and do what needs to be done for it to pass.

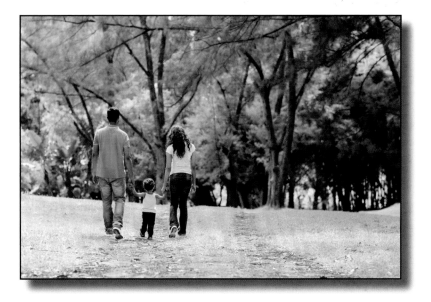

CHAPTER 2

16 Things to Do to Improve Your Cardiovascular Health and Fitness

The tips in this chapter are focused on the health of your cardiovascular system—your heart, lungs, blood vessels, and the rest of your internal plumbing that delivers blood and oxygen throughout your body.

#28: Find an Aerobic Activity You Enjoy

Imagine if there were a pill that dramatically improved nearly all aspects of your health with just a few doses per week, while having no real side effects. You'd be a fool not to take that pill, right?

That pill is regular aerobic exercise, in which you elevate your heart rate with sustained activity for twenty or more minutes at a time. Just a few hours a week of aerobic exercise significantly lowers your risk for cardiovascular disease, type 2 diabetes, and some types of cancer, and helps to control your weight and improves your mental state, among other benefits.

The issue for some people is that, instead of a pill, aerobic exercise is more like the proverbial castor oil—something you know you need, but lacking so much in appeal that it feels like a chore. When you feel like that, it can be hard to get yourself to exercise with the necessary frequency and consistency.

The key to overcoming that potential hurdle is to find an aerobic activity you enjoy doing. Then exercise will be more like play than the first syllable in the word "workout."

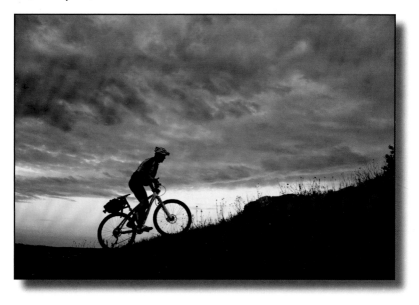

For me, that activity is running. In a physical sense, I enjoy the motion, the sense of exploration, being outside in all sorts of weather, the mood-improving endorphins, and the chance for quality time alone or with one or two good friends. Psychologically, running's simplicity, convenience, and rewarding of regularity suits my personality well. I like other activities such as hiking and cycling enough to happily do them, but nothing else speaks to me like running does.

My wife is a much more interesting person in an athletic sense. She enjoys regularly mixing activities, including cycling, running, Nordic skiing, kayaking, hiking, and snowshoeing. The variety keeps her more mentally engaged than concentrating on one activity, while the physical variation gives her the overall rather than sport-specific fitness she values. Her two favorites, cycling and skiing, appeal to her in part because she likes the changes in effort that topography naturally cause during a ride or ski. Her boring husband, on the other hand, is drawn to the steady rhythmic effort that marks a good run.

My point isn't that her way is better than mine, or vice versa. It's that we've been fortunate to find aerobic activities that we want to do, not that we feel like we have to do. As a result, it's easy for us to get the prescribed few hours a week of aerobic exercise, and then some, and reap the health benefits from doing things we'd want to do anyway.

What those activities are for you is up to you to discover. The keys are that they're appealing, enjoyable, suitable to your personality, and logistically practical for your life. That last point is key—you might discover that something like stand-up paddle boarding makes you feel fully alive, but if you can realistically do it only a few times a month, you'll need to find one or more supplementary activities to fill the gap.

While you're exploring activities, give each one at least a month of regular participation before deciding it's not for you. Even the simplest activity involves a learning curve before you're comfortable enough with it to decide if you enjoy it. That will be especially true if you're not in good cardiovascular shape. In that case, almost any activity is initially going to feel difficult. Wait until your fitness improves and you're past that hump before declaring a type of exercise isn't your thing.

Another stumbling block early on is finding the right effort level. Many people think that exercise is supposed to hurt to be effective. As a result, they wind up working too hard, getting out of breath quickly, and cutting their workout short. Aim for a perceived exertion of easy to moderate—your breathing and effort level should be greater than during a casual stroll, but you should be able to carry on a conversation.

#29: Come Up with Ways to Be More Active

You've probably heard that you should take at least 10,000 steps a day. Although this figure isn't an official recommendation from public health agencies such as the federal Centers for Disease Control and Prevention, it is an activity level that's been linked to health outcomes such as lower blood pressure and reduced blood sugar levels. And it makes an important point: most Americans aren't active enough.

By some estimates, the average American takes just more than 5,000 steps a day. Health researchers consider this to be a sedentary lifestyle, with all the negative health consequences that come with living that way. Bear in mind that this is a total for the entire day—not just planned exercise, but moving around the house, buying groceries, walking to the bathroom at work, and so on. And bear in mind that 5,000-plus steps per day is an average figure, meaning that many people are even less active once you account for people who are regular exercisers and/or active at work.

The average person used to be much more active. A study of Old Order Amish, whose lifestyle hasn't changed much since the nineteenth century, found that the average man in the community took more than 18,000 steps a day, and the average woman more than 14,000. An average adult takes about 2,000 steps per mile, so Amish adults get in roughly seven to nine miles per day of walking just through daily activities.

Over the last 150 years, much of the Amish's labor-intensive way of life has disappeared. In many ways, of course, that change has been welcome. But the health ramifications of labor-saving devices and environments that are engineered to prioritize automobiles are undeniable. We have reached the stage where most of us need to consciously add some labor back into our day.

As with many health-improvement measures, becoming more active doesn't mean making radical changes all at once. Many experts laud the 10,000-steps movement but say that if you're currently sedentary, your best bet is to start with small increases. If you use a step counter or other fitness tracker, try to take 1,000 more steps per day than you currently do. As that level of activity becomes seamlessly integrated into your lifestyle, add another 1,000 per day. Keep increasing in this manner until you're at 10,000 or more steps per day or meet the CDC's recommendation of at least 150 minutes of moderate activity per week.

Regular exercise is the obvious way to increase your activity level. But experts tell even hard-core athletes to avoid a routine of vigorous exercise followed by being sedentary for the rest of the day. A few simple ways to be more active: Take the stairs instead of elevators. (At the least, don't use the down elevator.) Keep walking on escalators. Don't use drive-throughs. Park at the far end of lots. Walk rather than drive when running errands near your home. (See item #30.) If you do drive, park in a central spot and go on foot to each of several stores. Go low-tech with your yard work. (See item #40.)

Convenience is killing us. Sometimes, short cuts are dead ends.

#30: Create a Car-Free Zone around Your Home

The next time you're in Manhattan, take a good look at the people walking down the street. Notice anything? That's right—not many of them are overweight, and almost none are obese.

While it's true that, on average, Americans who are better off financially tend to be slimmer, this phenomenon can't just be attributed to the relative wealth of Manhattanites. After all, many of the non-tourists you'll see live in other boroughs, or even outside of New York City.

One thing almost all these people share is that they regularly walk for transportation. Because of cost and convenience, New Yorkers walk when many other Americans drive—to and from work, when shopping, to get to public transportation, etc. Data collected by the fitness tracker manufacturer Fitbit show that, on average, New Yorkers accumulate more steps per day than residents of any other American city. Equally telling, unlike in other cities, New Yorkers walk almost the same amount in winter as they do in summer. They have to to go about their lives. Two unintended but felicitous consequences are a significant amount of heart-helping exercise and less incidence of overweight.

You can simulate the New York experience by creating a car-free zone around your home. Maybe it extends a mile in every direction. For trips within that zone, travel by foot or bike. Over time, you should accumulate enough extra movement in your day to impart health benefits.

Implementing this idea speaks to the concept we looked at in the previous item—that in modern society, we should sometimes choose to do things in other than the most convenient way. As with Manhattanites walking to the subway, for most of human history, daily life required people to use their bodies enough to produce health benefits. It now behooves many of us to consciously make some tasks a little more labor-intensive.

Having a car-free zone around your home can also change how you experience and think about your neighborhood. It's a way to slow down the pace of life in the area immediately around you, better giving your surroundings a feeling of refuge.

#31: Eat Dark Chocolate

This idea should be easy to sell you on: regularly eating small amounts of dark chocolate can lower your blood pressure and reduce your risk of having a stroke.

Karin Reid, PhD, is an Australian chocolate researcher who, in addition to having the world's coolest job, has found that cocoa products are effective in reducing blood pressure by 2 to 3 mm Hg in the short term. That's a significant enough reduction to improve cardiovascular health. Other long-term, large-scale studies have found an inverse relationship between chocolate consumption and the incidence of stroke. That is, those who reported eating the least amount of chocolate were more likely to have a stroke during the study period than those who said they ate more chocolate.

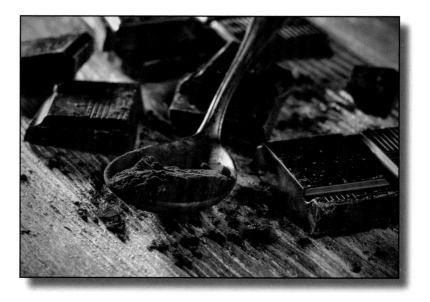

The mechanism for this apparent gift from nature is thought to be gut microbes metabolizing compounds in cocoa with names like catechin and epicatchin into smaller molecules with anti-inflammatory properties.

It's those compounds in cocoa (the flavonoids—see item #38) that provide the benefit. That means if you want to eat your way to better heart health, you'll need to eat dark chocolate that contains at least 50 percent cocoa. Milk chocolate won't get the job done.

Most people find dark chocolate with that high of a cocoa content to taste bitter without added fat and sugar. And once those latter items are added, dark chocolate becomes less of a superfood—a 100-gram bar of 85 percent dark chocolate contains 600 calories, 450 of which come from fat.

The good news is that research has found the cardiovascular benefits accrue at relatively low levels of consumption, even as little as six grams, or about a tenth of an ounce, per day. Reid says she eats one three- to six-gram piece of 50 to 70 percent dark chocolate daily.

#32: Control Your Reaction to Stress

Many of the things that cause us stress are external. We can't control whether a work project is dumped on us with a short deadline, the insurance company screwed up our medical billing, or the person in the car in front of us is texting away even though the light has turned green.

We can, however, control how we react to these events, and in doing so preserve our cardiovascular health.

Your body reacts to perceived stress by releasing the hormones adrenalin and cortisol and constricting your blood vessels. As a result, your heart rate and blood pressure increase. These fight-or-flight processes are helpful if your house is on fire or a bear is chasing you. They don't do you much good when your plane is delayed or a coworker fails to read an important message you sent.

Short-term reactions to stress haven't been shown to cause long-term high blood pressure. But if you're having these reactions three times an hour, day after day, you're certainly not improving your health. It's reasonable to say chronic stress can harm your overall wellness.

There are two key ways to limit stress. First, find ways to alter your reaction. The fight-or-flight response may be hard-wired into us but is neither helpful nor appropriate in much of modern life. Learn to override that response. Analyze the situation: Is it really that bad? Is there anything I can do to change it without confrontation? Is it worth losing control of my emotions over? Is it likely to end soon even if I don't do anything? Remind yourself that having a stressful reaction makes the person causing you to feel that way that much more in control of you. On a practical level, do something to stop the stressful reaction. Breathe deeply and calmly, hum a favorite song, look away, go for a walk, or put on headphones. Do something to break your typical reaction to the trigger.

The second solution is to avoid situations that you know will stress you, even once you've gotten better in how you react to these situations. Few of us are Zen master enough not to be bothered by things like rush-hour traffic or crowds of holiday shoppers. Most of us know people who have a way of getting under our skin. When possible, remove yourself from predictable sources of stress. Along those same lines, don't create known stressful situations, such as putting off work projects or your tax returns until the last minute, or getting to the airport too soon before your flight.

There's another aspect to controlling your reaction to stress. During sustained stressful periods, it's common to turn to things like cigarettes, alcohol, tubes of cookie dough, etc. It's easy to justify a just-this-once mentality when you're looking for immediate relief. But whatever aid they might provide is temporary and won't do away with the cause of your stress, while worsening your health.

#33: Get a Petable Pet

If you've ever felt better after spending time with a dog instead of people, you're not necessarily misanthropic. You probably just experienced the research-backed benefits of certain types of pets.

In one fascinating experiment, researchers measured people's blood pressure while the subjects petted, talked to, and looked at a dog, and also while the people talked to (but didn't pet!) the researchers. The subjects' blood pressure was lowest when they petted a dog and highest while they talked with the researchers. When the people talked to or looked at a dog, their blood pressure was still lower than when they talked to a human. The researchers concluded that the touch element of the encounter somehow triggered the most beneficial blood-pressure response. This finding suggests that dogs and cats are better for your cardiovascular health than, say, goldfish.

There are other ways that dogs in particular have been linked with improved health. Several studies have found that dog owners tend to be more active than non-dog owners, and that this greater activity level is associated with a better cardiovascular profile and lower weight. Walking the dog once or twice a day is another great example of how something simple, non-strenuous, and (usually) enjoyable done for practical purposes can have unintended but significant health benefits.

Along those lines, as anyone who has ever walked a puppy in the presence of strangers can attest, dogs are a great way to get humans who would otherwise ignore one another to converse. Short, casual social interactions are a boost to mental health by virtue of reducing feelings of isolation. Some psychologists recommend dog ownership for people with mild to moderate depression, both for the companionship and uncomplicated love the animal provides and the likely greater social connections the pooch will lead to.

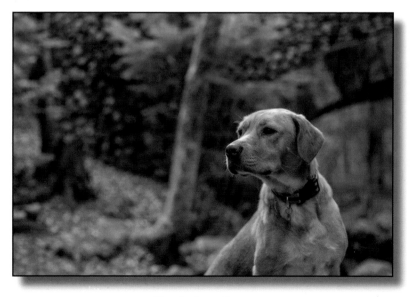

Photo by Stacey Cramp

#34: Know Your Heart Rate

An elevated heart rate can be the sign that one of several undesirable things is going on in your body. Possibilities include high blood pressure, coronary artery disease, heart muscle disease, tumors, and infections.

Knowing your normal heart rate will help you better decide if something is amiss. Your heart rate varies throughout the day, depending on many factors, including body position, stress level, caffeine intake, and recent activity. Your lowest typical pulse, when you've been sitting or lying still for a while, is known as your resting heart rate. It should be relatively stable from day to day.

The best time to get a good baseline figure for your normal resting heart rate is when you wake. Lie still until you feel calm. (This might take longer if you wake to an alarm.) Without too much pressure, place one or two fingers on the inside of your wrist or the side of your neck to find your pulse. Count the number of heartbeats in fifteen seconds and multiply that figure by four to get your resting heart rate. Repeat this exercise over several mornings to get an idea of what's typical.

If you feel like your heart rate has increased recently, try to measure it as above, when you're likely to get the lowest reading for the day. A one-day bump probably isn't cause for concern—poor sleep, dehydration, stress from work, and other temporary situations can cause that. Similarly, if you're clearly sick, then don't worry about an elevated heart rate. If, however, you notice a repeated increase over your norm and can't identify an obvious reason, seek medical attention.

#35: Eat Whole Grains

Large-scale studies consistently show that people who regularly eat whole-grain foods have a lower risk of developing many chronic conditions, including coronary artery disease and cardiovascular disease. A diet high in whole grains is also associated with lower cholesterol levels and less incidence of cancer, diabetes, respiratory diseases, and infectious diseases. In study periods of various lengths, people who eat a lot of whole grains are less likely to die than those who don't.

The fiber in whole grains is thought to play a large role in their heart-health benefits. Fiber is believed to attach itself to cholesterol particles and help remove them from your system. By promoting a feeling of fullness, fiber is also credited with helping people stay at a healthy weight. Being overweight is an independent risk factor for

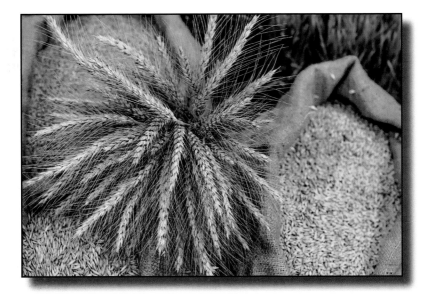

some diseases. In addition, whole grains are a good source of many nutrients that have their own health benefits.

Refined grains, in which the bran and germ have been stripped away, contain little of the fiber and nutrients of whole grains.

Some studies have found a benefit from adding just one serving of whole grains to your daily diet. Greater benefits appear to occur at around three daily servings. Some common examples of one serving of whole grains are one piece of whole-wheat bread, half a cup of cooked whole-grain pasta or brown rice, and one whole-wheat tortilla.

For many people, obtaining these servings can be accomplished by replacing a current refined grain product—such as white bread, white pasta, or white rice—with its whole-grain counterpart. In addition to whole wheat, readily available sources of whole grains include brown rice, whole oats, wild rice, whole-grain barley, and popcorn. (Yes, popcorn!)

#36: Drink Wine (in Moderation)

People have strong feelings about alcohol, and for good reason. Excessive alcohol consumption leads to problems ranging from liver disease and traffic fatalities to neurological conditions and ruined relationships. There are many people who are better off living an alcohol-free life. For people who can enjoy alcohol at light to moderate levels of consumption without risk of becoming a heavier drinker, there's good evidence of cardiovascular benefits, especially from red wine.

When the results of several studies are pooled, light to moderate alcohol consumption is associated with a 20-percent lower risk of developing coronary artery disease or having a stroke. The same level of consumption is associated with about a 30-percent lower risk of having a heart attack. It's thought that alcohol helps to maintain healthy blood vessels, thereby lowering the risk of arteries clogging.

Although the evidence is equivocal, it appears that red wine might confer additional benefits over beverages such as beer or white wine. It's thought that chemical compounds in red wine known as polyphenols (see item #38) contribute to blood-vessel maintenance independent of that caused by alcohol.

The amounts in these studies are in the range of one or two five-ounce glasses of wine a few to several days per week. The takeaway is that if you enjoy drinking this amount, you can further enjoy it knowing you're helping your heart. But more is definitely not better. And health experts agree that people who don't currently drink shouldn't start just to get the heart-health benefits.

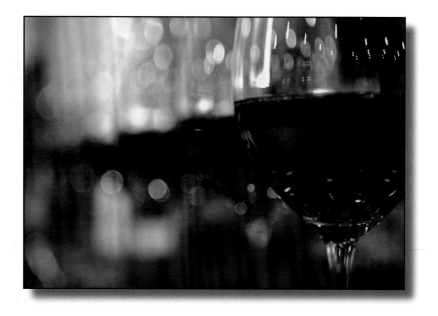

#37: Eat Nuts

"A handful of nuts a day" lacks the poetic pizzazz of the daily-apple version, but it contains at least as much medical validity.

Consider the findings of a study that looked at diet and disease in 118,000 people over a thirty-year period. It found that frequent nut consumption was associated with a lower risk of all-cause and disease-specific death. Compared to people who didn't eat nuts, those who ate a one-ounce serving of nuts seven or more times a week had a 20-percent lower risk of all-cause death (i.e., they were less likely to die for whatever reason during the long period studied). Eating nuts five or more times per week was also associated with a 25-percent lower risk of cardiovascular-related death and a 29-percent lower risk of heart disease. The study also found

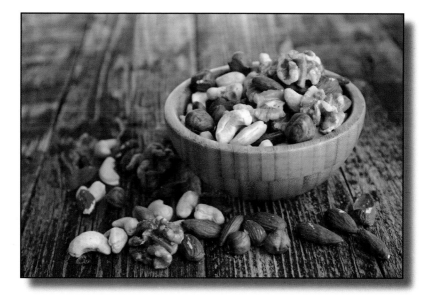

an 11-percent lower risk of cancer-related death and a 24-percent lower risk of death from respiratory disease among regular nut eaters.

In the study, one-ounce servings of peanuts and tree nuts (almonds, pecans, walnuts, pine nuts, etc.) had similar effects on lowering mortality. There are about twenty to twenty-five almonds, and fifteen to twenty peanuts or cashews, in a one-ounce serving.

Nuts are dense with vitamins, minerals, protein, and antioxidants. They are also higher in fat than most foods touted as disease-fighting, but it's thought that the unsaturated fat in them helps to lower, not raise, cholesterol levels.

There's even evidence that regular nut consumption might not hurt, and could even aid, people watching their weight. One study found that the caloric value of almonds has been overestimated by 32 percent. It based its calculations on analyzing waste products when nuts were eaten as part of a mixed diet, in contrast to the traditional method of assigning caloric values, which analyzes food in isolation. The newer method, of course, more closely aligns with how things happen in the real world.

Another factor in nuts' favor for dieters: in one study, subjects who ate dry-roasted almonds—either with breakfast or lunch, or as a morning or afternoon snack—curbed their appetite without gaining weight. The snackers had their almonds two hours after a meal and two hours before their next meal. All the nut eaters in the study had a one-and-a-half ounce serving per day. Their total caloric intake didn't increase, and they didn't gain weight during the month-long study. According to the researchers, the subjects adjusted their diet because they didn't feel as hungry between meals and during meals.

#38: Eat Berries

Nuts' partner in the common pairing also appears to have heart-health benefits, with no concern whatsoever about its caloric content.

In one study of more than 90,000 women, those who ate three or more servings of berries each week were found to have a significantly lower risk of heart attack over an eighteen-year follow-up period. Another study of almost 2,000 men found that, over a twelve-year follow-up period, those who ate the most berries had a significantly lower rate of death from heart disease than those who ate the least amount of berries. Such evidence isn't isolated and has led to berries being included in most health experts' recommendations for a heart-healthy diet.

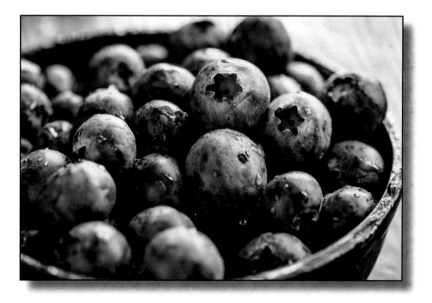

Berries are high in flavonoids, one type of the micronutrient family known as polyphenols. These substances are increasingly believed to have cancer-preventive and anti-inflammatory benefits. There's even evidence that berries can help aging brains. One review of studies on the matter concluded that eating a lot of berries helps to preserve neural communication in the brain, thereby lessening the cognitive decline often associated with aging. It's this apparent ability to lower your risk for major diseases that always lands berries on lists of superfoods.

Flavonoids give many plants, including berries, their bright color. Variety in your diet is always a good idea, and that includes the matter of color. Choosing fruits and vegetables of a broad range of colors should increase your consumption of flavonoids and lower your risk of some diseases.

#39: Drink Tea

Chalk up another one for flavonoids, which we looked at in the previous item. In the case of tea, the flavonoids present are thought to help lower inflammation and improve vascular health, resulting in less build-up of plaque in your arteries. Arterial plaque is responsible for what's commonly called clogged arteries. Plaque can slow blood flow or, more dangerous, rupture, resulting in a blood clot that causes a heart attack or stroke.

Research on regular tea drinkers has found that they may be less likely to have heart attacks and strokes. There's also evidence supporting tea's role in lowering blood pressure and LDL ("bad") cholesterol levels.

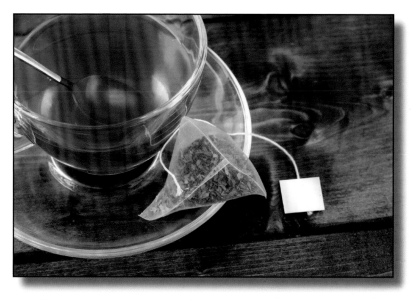

The tea in question comes from the plant *Camellia sinensis*. The leaves of this evergreen shrub are used in all black and green teas. Herbal teas, such as chamomile, rooibos, or ginger, are called teas because their method of preparation, steeping, is what's done with black or green tea. While these herbal teas may have health benefits, and are enjoyable, they don't contain the flavonoids found in the leaves of *Camellia sinensis*. Because of differences in how green and black teas are made, green tea contains more flavonoids.

#40: Care for Your Yard the Low-Tech Way

It's not only possible, but better for you to gather leaves, mow the lawn, and clear snow with human-powered rather than gas-powered tools. I live in Maine, and I can vouch for the fact that it's possible to get through the winter with just a shovel.

This gets back to an idea introduced earlier—modern life has made it so easy to avoid activity that we need to find ways to reintroduce it. Put another way, the existence of a gas-powered gadget shouldn't automatically make it the default means of doing a task. Mowing by hand, raking leaves, and shoveling snow are exactly the types of moderate-intensity activities that contributed to earlier generations' better health. They'll get your heart rate up and exercise large muscles throughout your body. Raking and bagging leaves burns an estimated 350 to 450 calories per hour, a little more than an hour of brisk walking for most people. Shoveling snow can burn up to 600 calories an hour, close to what a lot of people expend to run six miles.

These devices can harm your health other than by reducing your activity level. A typical leaf blower operates at a volume of eighty-five or

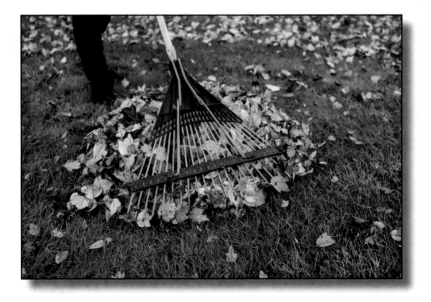

more decibels, louder than the threshold at which hearing is harmed. The same device is also an emissions nightmare—a leaf blower with the common two-stroke engine pollutes as much in half an hour as a pick-up truck does driving across the United States one and a half times. And while you're blowing leaves, you're also dispersing allergens, pesticides, and other particulates that can lead to health problems.

An irony is that these devices save you labor but might not save you time. Picture someone with a leaf blower slowly ushering their pile of leaves along. You don't have to be a Luddite to agree that the leaves could be raked much more quickly. Similarly, I regularly clear snow from my driveway in less time than my neighbor does with a snow blower.

One more way that low-tech yard care can improve your health: the neighbors won't throw something at your head for ruining their weekend afternoon with your leaf blower.

#41: Take a Walk after Dinner

After Thanksgiving dinner, while some people collapse on the couch in a food coma, others head outside for a leisurely stroll. Even people who are usually sedentary will instinctively walk around the block.

Trust those instincts. Walking after your largest meal of the day has important benefits in addition to the calorie-burning and fitness-improving ones that accrue at all times.

Research has found that a brief walk (fifteen to twenty minutes) lessens the spike in blood sugar levels that typically occurs after a large meal. Large rises and falls in blood sugar levels can increase your risk for cardiovascular disease and are particularly dangerous for diabetics and pre-diabetics. At least one study has found that a shorter walk after a large meal tempers blood sugar spikes better than a longer walk before eating.

Walking after dinner is an example of a practice whose benefits transcend one type of health. In addition to the above, a post-meal ambulation has been shown to aid in digestion (the likely explanation for why people are more inclined to engage in the practice on Thanksgiving). In one study that compared following a meal with a walk to a post-dinner caffeinated beverage or alcoholic digestif, only the walk increased the rate at which food emptied from the stomach.

And yet another benefit: in another study, people who delayed having dessert until after going on a short walk ate about half the amount of chocolate compared to when they indulged immediately after the main course.

#42: Jump Rope

Michael Joyner, MD, a health researcher at the Mayo Clinic, has stood before a conference of fellow experts and touted a fitness device that's effective, inexpensive, portable, and convenient. Then, with the attendees expecting to see the latest digital gadget, Joyner pulls out a jump rope.

Once you (re)learn how to do it, jumping rope can provide a great cardiovascular workout in a short amount of time. When you get a good rhythm going, your heart rate will be at the desired level that is high enough to produce the desired benefits but not so high that you can't sustain the activity. (For most adults, continuing to coordinate the motion of jumping rope is what will first bring them to a halt. But the aerobic benefits will still accrue if you resume jumping rope almost immediately.)

Jumping rope at a good but sustainable effort level can burn about the same number of calories per minute as running. Of course, it's unlikely you'll do a straight thirty minutes of jumping rope like you might running, cycling, or using an elliptical machine. A good whole-body workout alternates five minutes of jumping rope with a minute of body-weight exercises, such as push-ups and planks (see Chapter 3), then immediately back to jumping rope.

Jumping rope has other benefits. As we'll see in the next chapter, weight-bearing activities such as jumping rope help to build and maintain strong bones. Jumping rope will also improve your balance, which we'll also look at in the next chapter, and what's known as neuromuscular coordination, or how well your brain, nervous system, and muscles work together. Better balance and coordination can have huge payoffs in daily life, especially with age, as they help you to avoid falls and generally better navigate your physical environment.

Joyner's advocacy of jumping rope makes a larger point: simplicity often means an activity is easier to do on a regular basis than a supposedly more advanced or more effective type of workout.

#43: Wear Compression Socks on Airplanes

With long security lines, smaller seats, checked-bag fees, and other features, airline travel these days is often irksome. Don't let it also be unhealthful.

Sitting with little change of position for a long time increases your risk of deep vein thrombosis, a type of blood clot. The clots can damage the veins they form in or, more dangerously, can break loose and travel through the bloodstream. In that case, they put you at risk for pulmonary embolism, a blockage of a blood vessel in your lungs. Pulmonary embolism can damage your lungs and in some cases can be fatal.

Deep vein thrombosis can develop in your legs, arms, or torso, but are most likely to occur in your legs during air travel. A good precautionary measure is to wear compression socks, which, by applying external pressure to muscles, improves the flow of blood in veins back to the heart. Better circulation, in turn, lessens swelling and pooling of blood in your feet and lower legs.

You might think about compression socks primarily as something worn by older people with vascular problems, but they're increasingly favored by high-level athletes and available in styles and colors other than hospital white. Graduated compression socks, which apply reduced pressure from the foot up the leg, are believed to be more effective at reducing swelling during air travel.

You can further reduce your risk of deep vein thrombosis by leaving your seat when you can. (If possible, book an aisle seat to increase your chance of escape.) Walk the aisle and do light stretching and exercises such as squats in the area by the bathrooms. If you're seat-bound for more than an hour, increase foot and lower-leg circulation with in-place exercises such as twirling your feet in circles and pretending that you're pressing on and releasing the gas pedal in a car.

CHAPTER 3

24 Things to Do to Improve Your Muscular/Skeletal Health and Fitness

In this chapter, we'll look at how to keep your muscles and bones strong and functioning well, so that your quality of movement is high and your risk of pain and injury is low.

#44: Set Up Your Workstation Properly

In Chapter 1, we looked at why you should limit the amount of time per day you sit. When you do sit, try to do so in the least harmful way.

Slouching rounds your lower back, rounds your shoulder, and thrusts your head forward. This posture increases the load on your spine and strains the muscles of your upper back, shoulders and neck. The potential cascade of compensatory pain and discomfort throughout your body is nearly infinite.

The key to mitigating sitting while you work is to keep a straight spine. According to Daniel Frey, DPT, author of *The Runner's Guide to a Healthy Core,* a straight spine while sitting isn't synonymous with a vertical spine. If you work on a laptop computer or perform work on top of your desk, such as processing paperwork, leaning forward may be better, Frey says. Sit toward the front of your chair instead of using the back support. Bend your feet underneath you slightly so that your knees are lower to the ground than your hips.

If you use a monitor instead of a laptop screen, position it at eye level. It should be close enough that you don't have to move your head forward to read, but far enough away to lessen the glare.

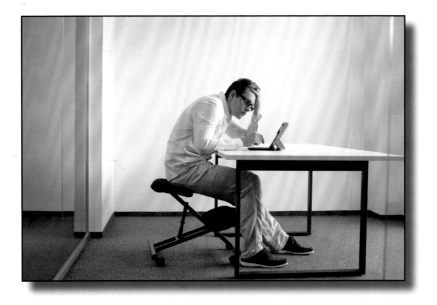

(See item #18 about computers and eyesight.) For most people, that means having the monitor twenty to twenty-six inches away. If you use a monitor, your spine will be better positioned if it is closer to vertical, Frey says. He recommends holding a book on top of your head. If it stays in place, your head is in a good position.

Keep your wrists straight to help them relax. Don't rest them on your desk or the area in front of the keyboard on a laptop. If you use a mouse, keep your hand on it only when you need to move the cursor or click. Otherwise, remove your hand to relax it.

Try not to sit in one position for more than twenty minutes at a time. If you're unable to stand and continue working, take short breaks, even if to just walk around your desk or do a few squats. Kneel on one or both knees briefly to stretch the muscles in the top front of your legs. While sitting, squeeze your butt cheeks toward each other for a count of five, relax, and repeat a few times. Shift most of your weight onto one sit bone for a minute, shift to the other for a minute, then return to normal sitting. Place a small rolled towel behind your lower back. Keep coming up with ways to change position and keep your back, butt, and leg muscles activated and well fed with blood.

#45: Stand While You Work

The previous item was about how to sit in the least harmful way. Note I said "least harmful" instead of "most healthful." As we've seen, extensive sitting is bad for many aspects of your health.

An increasing number of office workers are opting to work some or all of the day standing. You could do worse financially than to have a stake in a company that makes standing desks; sales continue to rise as the consequences of sitting become more known.

There are two schools of thought on the best set-up. One advocates having a workstation at which you can only stand, so that you won't be tempted to sit. The other recommends an adjustable workstation, so that you can alternate sitting or standing. The standing-only method is certainly better long-term and doesn't mean you can't have a chair elsewhere in your office.

Early on, most people will do best to gradually transition to standing while working. Start with one hour in the morning and one hour in the afternoon. Your feet, calf muscles, and butt will be some of the main complainers as you adjust. Over time, add other standing sessions of an hour or less. Fatigue in newly engaged body parts is acceptable; pain isn't. The longer you've been chairbound, the more time you should allow to get used to

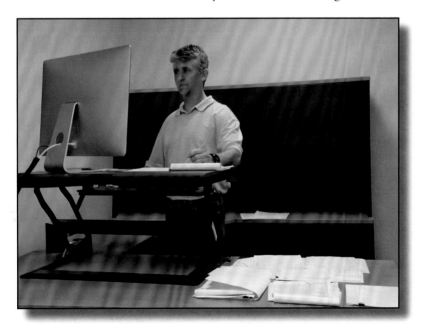

this new way of working. As with many new health-improvement projects, your chances of long-term success will be greater if you patiently progress in small increments rather than go all in from day one.

If your company won't provide you a standing desk and you're unable to afford one, see if you can get away with an improvised variable desk. For example, alternate a traditional sitting set-up with putting your laptop on top of a milk crate or small bench, and placing that item on your desk.

Consider getting a mat, such as you might see grocery cashiers use, to stand on. A softer but not squishy platform will lessen foot and leg fatigue.

If you're unable to integrate standing into your main work, make use of other opportunities to sit less. Stand during phone calls, when reading print materials, while brainstorming, and any other time you're not tied to your laptop or other deskbound machinery.

If you're going to stand more while working, you need to be in the right shoes. (Hint: not heels.) See items #50 and #51 below for more on healthful footwear.

As a cashier could tell you, standing doesn't replace the need for regular movement. Continue to incorporate regular breaks and changes of bodily position into your workday.

#46: Stand Up Straight

Whether you're at a desk or elsewhere, good posture while standing relieves the load on your skeleton, lessens muscular strains, and reduces your risk of joint pain because forces are spread more evenly throughout your body rather than overly absorbed by your knees and hips.

In good standing posture, your head, shoulders, hips, and ankles are aligned. Your eyes are facing forward, and your jawbone is parallel to the ground. (Chin up!) Your weight is evenly distributed between your left and right sides. Your weight is also evenly distributed from the back to the front of your feet, rather than concentrated on your heels or the balls of your feet.

Most of us will find standing like this a challenge. Try this: stand against a wall with your heels, pelvis, back, shoulders, and head touching the surface of the wall. This is good standing posture. Now take a few steps forward. Are you still in that position? Probably not. Your head probably moved forward, your shoulders probably rounded, and you probably shifted some of your weight forward so that it was no longer evenly distributed throughout your feet.

One challenge that we long-time slumpers have is holding our shoulders correctly. Check on their position frequently when you stand. Lightly pull them backward and down; feel your shoulder blades move down your back. Envision that your shoulders are low, level, and relaxed, and in line with your hips. Without straining your neck or shoulders, visualize creating more distance between the tops of your shoulders and the bottom of your head.

Head position is often another big challenge. Once you're holding your shoulders correctly, move your head so that your ears are lined up with your shoulders. Notice how this moves your head back, your chin up, and your gaze forward. Reacquainting yourself with this position can feel odd after years of looking down at a computer screen or phone. Periodically imagine that you're trying to balance a book on the top of your head. If you realize it would slide down the front or off one side, reposition your head.

When in doubt, return to the wall position to remind yourself what proper standing alignment feels like.

#47: Try Not to Cross Your Legs When You Sit

We saw earlier in this chapter why and how to sit with good posture. But, you know, things happen, and especially early in the process of relearning how to sit properly, it's common to find that you've reverted to old habits. One position you might find yourself in is sitting with one leg crossed over the other.

As soon as you notice you're sitting like this, uncross your legs and put both feet on the ground. There are three good reasons to take this action.

First, sitting with your legs crossed makes your hips uneven. That's never good. In the short term, the twist that comes from sitting with your legs crossed can lead to muscular tension from your lower back on up to your neck. Over time, frequently being in a crossed-leg position could cause your pelvis to shift such that you're always out of alignment. This will alter your gait and can lead to compensatory changes throughout your body. For example, if your pelvis becomes even slightly tilted to the left, your hip and leg muscles on that side could develop low-grade chronic strain from working harder to stabilize your hips when you walk and do other movements.

You may have noticed after sitting with crossed legs that the foot of the crossed leg feels tingly or "asleep." That's probably because sitting in that position impinged on the crossed leg's peroneal nerve, which runs behind the knee down the outer leg into the foot. Repeatedly compromising the nerve in this fashion can damage it, leading to loss of some foot and ankle function.

Your heart also doesn't appreciate whatever temporary comfort you might derive from sitting with your legs crossed. The position makes it harder to move blood from your feet and legs back up to the heart, resulting in temporarily elevated blood pressure. As with the peroneal nerve compression, the blood pressure spike can be undone by getting out of the crossed-leg position. But also as with the peroneal nerve, regular short-term episodes can accumulate to long-term negative effect.

Not crossing your legs when you sit is the sort of thing you might need to be mindful of at first but that will occur less as you move toward better practices.

#48: Keep Your Body Aligned When You're Driving

Research on professional drivers has found high incidences of lower back pain (65 percent), neck pain (43 percent), and shoulder pain (40 percent). There are indications that vibrations from the vehicle contribute to some of these woes, but the biggest factor is the difficulty in maintaining good posture when behind the wheel. When you consider how much some of us drive, it's obvious this isn't a problem only for the pros.

That your body experiences driving as a form of insult makes intuitive sense—not many people spring out of the car ready for a game of pick-up basketball. More common is a slow rise out of the seat, perhaps with an assist from your arms because your legs don't feel up to the task, then a sort of John Wayne cowboy sideways stagger for at least a few steps while your lower back, butt, and hamstrings come back to life.

There are several things you can do to lessen the toll that driving takes on your body. Don't recline your seat more than a few degrees beyond 90 degrees. Keep the seat flat so that your hips are close to the height of your knees. Sit with as much of your thighs supported by the seat as possible. A small towel rolled under your hips or behind your lower back can help to maintain good alignment.

Also, try not to let large muscles such as your hamstrings and glutes be idle for too long. Obviously, for safety's sake you're limited in how much you can move around, but occasional subtle shifts in position can help to keep these muscles from falling asleep (more accurately, getting a diminished blood supply). One really good trick: every fifteen minutes, contract your butt muscles. Imagine trying to squeeze your butt cheeks toward each other. Contract, hold for a few seconds, relax, and repeat a few times.

Finally, check periodically that you're maintaining your initial good posture: when you first get in the car, sit with good alignment and move the rearview mirror so that it provides a clear view of what's behind you while you're in this position. Throughout your drive, when you check the rearview mirror, look to see if the view is the same as when you started. If it's not, you're slouching. Sit back up to obtain your original view.

#49: Sleep Well

When you consider that you spend close to one-third of your life sleeping, it makes sense that the position you sleep in and other aspects of your time in bed affect how your body feels and operates.

The biggest matter for most people in this regard is whether their sleep position strains their back. Experts advise sleeping in a position that maintains the natural curve of your lower back. For many people, this means sleeping on their side, with the knees drawn slightly toward the chest. Sleeping on your back is even better for maintaining a neutral spine but can lead to more interruptions while you sleep, such as from snoring or other breathing matters when you're congested from a cold or allergies. Sleeping on your stomach, in contrast, increases strain on your back and can cause neck pain from having your head turned to one side for several hours.

Of course, it's easier to consciously change your position for something like how you sit at work compared to how you sleep. Depending on in which position you naturally spend the most time, you can make things easier on your spine and neck by choosing the appropriate pillow. If you mostly sleep on your back, use a soft pillow so that your head isn't propped up too much. If you have frequent back pain, try placing a second pillow under your knees to help maintain a slight curve in your lower back. If you mostly sleep on your side, use a thick pillow so that your head and neck stay better aligned with your spine. If you have frequent back pain, place a second pillow between your legs.

If you can't help but to sleep on your stomach, use as thin a pillow as possible, or none, to better keep your head and neck aligned. Stomach sleepers who have back pain can get some relief by placing a second pillow under the pelvis and lower abdomen.

#50: Wear Flat Shoes

Shoes with heels bring to mind two Latin phrases. First, *De gustibus non est disputandum*—in matters of taste, there can be no disputes. If you think wearing heels looks good, I can't tell you otherwise. But in the context of this book, I can tell you the other Latin phrase, *Caveat emptor*—let the buyer beware. Stylish or not, shoes with heels are bad for your body.

Consider a study that measured calf muscle length and Achilles tendon agility in women who regularly wear high heels versus women who don't. The heel wearers had calf muscles that were about 12 percent shorter than those of the non-heel wearers. The heel wearers' Achilles tendons were more than 10 percent

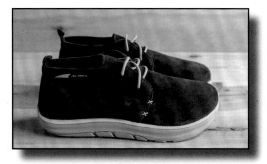

Photo by Stacey Cramp

more rigid than those of the non-heel wearers. As a result, the heel wearers had significantly less range of motion in their ankles.

A different study showed how these sorts of structural changes have functional implications. Researchers gathered two groups: one made up of women who had worn heels of at least 5 centimeters (a little less than 2 inches) for forty hours a week for at least two years, and the other made up of women who had worn heels for less than ten hours a week. While the women walked over level ground, the researchers measured ankle and knee motion and lower leg muscle activity. The heel wearers had measurable increases in fascial strain and muscle activity compared to the other group. Their history of wearing heels for much of the workweek had negatively altered their basic walking mechanics.

Heels also tip your pelvis forward, leading to some of the same alignment problems as those caused by poor sitting posture, including lower back strain and weakening of the powerful muscles on your backside.

Running shoe companies and other active-wear brands are among the leaders in making flat shoes that can be worn in professional settings. Merrell, Altra, VivoBarefoot, and others have taken the design principles behind their barefoot-style athletic shoes and successfully applied them to loafers, lace-up flats, desert boots, and the like.

If heels are unavoidable in your profession, do the best you can to minimize the time you spend in them, such as wearing other shoes while commuting and taking the heels off when you know you'll be at your desk for a while.

Also, go barefoot or wear socks and/or slippers around the house. Why wear shoes inside? Shedding them will not only help your body, but also keep your floors and carpets clean.

#51: Wear Shoes That Fit Your Feet, Not Vice Versa

Hopefully I've convinced you to reconsider wearing shoes with heels. Now let's move on to other aspects of daily footwear.

Try this: If you're wearing shoes, take one off and line up your bare foot with your shod foot. What do you see?

Ideally, you'll see that your bare foot widens continually from the heel to the base of the toes. The arch of that foot is engaged, helping to distribute your weight over the foot. Your toes of that foot are probably spread out, and all of them are probably touching the ground.

Now compare that to your shod foot. A typical shoe will be almost the same width from the back to the base of your toes. At that point it will probably taper, either to a half circle at the top or, worse, a point. If you were to X-ray your shod foot, you'd probably see your toes bunched together, perhaps even overlapping as they accommodate the shape of the shoe.

As we saw when looking at the effects of high heels, over time your body will make undesirable adjustments when the natural movement of your feet is hindered or constrained. This will affect how you walk and stand, with ramifications for the muscles and bones throughout your body.

That being the case, it's important that the shoes you wear most often are in harmony with your feet. Unfortunately, that's not always our primary consideration. While we might obsess over the shoes we wear a few hours a week for gym workouts or running, we often pick shoes for daily living based on color and design, even though we wear these shoes for many more hours per week than workout shoes.

For starters, look for shoes that closely match the shape of your foot. They should be widest where your foot is widest. Your toes should be able to splay, much as if you were barefoot.

Shoes should also be flexible. While rigid shoes like work boots are sometimes necessary, most of us don't need to wear such shoes for work. A shoe that allows your arch to work naturally as a powerful spring allows for better shock absorption. When your foot is confined in a stiff, rigid shoe and your arch is unable to do its job, the joints in your legs and spine are placed under increased load.

Finally, look for shoes that are low to the ground. More distance between the bottom of your foot and the ground—even if the shoe is relatively flat—means less ability for your feet to sense the ground and react quickly to its surroundings. In the short term, this can increase your risk of trips or falls. Over time it can alter your balance and ability to make use of the information your feet are meant to transmit to the rest of your body.

#52: Walk Like a Runway Model

Phil Wharton is a world-renowned physiotherapist who wrote the foreword for this book. He treats top-level athletes from several sports as well as everyday people whose bodily woes are affecting their quality of life.

No matter the person's background or physical complaint, one of the first things they'll do when they see Wharton is walk across the room while he watches. This quick assessment tells Wharton much about whether the person properly performs one of the basic human movements.

Picture an old man walking. One foot is picked up, thrust out ahead and then slapped back down. Most of the rest of his body is rigid and uninvolved. He moves as if being pulled forward and attempting with each step not to fall over.

Now picture a runway model walking. Her hips and butt are engaged, propelling her forward while her arms move in synch with her legs. She moves in a tall, graceful way with good posture.

Most of the people Wharton sees, even highly accomplished athletes, walk more like the old person than the runway model. This stems from what Wharton calls "glutes in hibernation," which means that your posterior chain—the strong muscles along your backside—has become weak and tight from misuse. (The amount of sitting most of us do is a leading cause.) As a result, the body compensates by shifting tasks like walking from backside muscles elsewhere. An extreme example is the old person above, who walks by using the hip flexors in the front of the legs to lift one foot at a time and place it a few inches ahead.

There are two compelling reasons to relearn how to walk properly. First, it's always good to use your body as it evolved to be used. Walking by pushing with your butt muscles instead of pulling with your thigh muscles will help to reactivate your posterior chain, leading to more power and efficiency in your daily activities. Second, walking properly leads to better alignment, which in turn results in more even distribution of forces on your body and fewer back, shoulder, and neck aches and pains.

The next time you're walking down the street, take a moment to assess your gait. If it feels like your hips are rigid and most of the motion is coming from the front of your legs, visualize a runway model. As you begin to take a step forward, contract the glute muscle of that leg. Notice how doing so engages your pelvis as you start to push forward. The opposite arm will swing forward. Land not on your heel, as if you're braking, but on your midfoot, which will help to propel you forward. Your shoulders and hips will be aligned, in contrast to your being bent forward at the waist, as often occurs in the old-man walk.

Wharton calls this "a proud walk." Indeed, at first it can feel almost like you're strutting. You might have to remind yourself that it's okay to be presenting yourself to the world in a new way. Eventually you'll lose whatever self-consciousness might come from walking like this.

Start by interspersing segments of runway-model walking with your normal gait. Over time keep increasing the amount of your new powerful walking style until it becomes your norm.

#53: Walk Backward

Watch children play, and you'll see them moving easily in all directions. Most adults, however, have but one orientation they can confidently manage—forward. They've lost the functional dexterity that used to come naturally. If that's you—if moving any way but straight ahead is challenging—you should regularly do small amounts of backward walking.

Relearning how to move in more than one direction has significant benefits. In research on people recovering from knee injuries, people who did both backward and forward walking as part of their rehab had greater gains in quadriceps, hamstring, calf, and shin muscle strength compared to people who did only forward walking. The unfamiliar motion of walking backward challenged the front and back leg muscles enough that they responded by getting stronger. In contrast, the accustomed forward gait wasn't nearly as much of a stress. This is good for getting through daily activities without injury and undue fatigue, but not so good for getting stronger.

Another big benefit is that the relative lack of visual cues when you're walking backward helps to improve your balance and coordination. (See item #62 to learn how much we rely on seeing to maintain our balance.) You might also be inspired to try backward walking when you hear it burns more calories than forward walking.

Start with small amounts of backward walking in a setting you're familiar with. For example, go backward the last couple hundred yards as you approach your home on a walk around the block or from a store. Look back occasionally to make sure your path is free of obstacles and traffic. Other good options are going up and down stairs backward, and mixing in some backward motion when walking on a treadmill or using an elliptical machine.

#54: Stretch Regularly

Remember our old man walking in item #52? Let's say he's making his way down the sidewalk when he spots a dollar bill on the ground.

Picture him trying to pick it up. Now imagine a child who sees the bill and moves to claim it. What do you see?

For the old man, you probably visualized a stiff, unsuccessful attempt to bend forward, while the child quickly and effortlessly scooped up the bill. The difference between the two is largely because of differences in flexibility and mobility. Flexibility has to do with the length of a muscle—what's its maximum stretch point? Mobility has to do with the suppleness of a muscle—what's its ability to move freely within the range dictated by its length? Together, flexibility and mobility determine how freely you can move. In the next item, we'll look at the best ways to increase mobility. Here we'll look at how to build flexibility.

You might be most familiar with stretching as something to do before working out. And when you think stretching, you probably think of what's known as static stretching, or moving into a position that stretches a muscle and holding the stretch for a while. Static stretching as traditionally practiced has largely fallen out of favor with active people. Stretching in this way before activity, when muscles are cold, has been shown to reduce muscular power during the ensuing activity. It can also produce what's known as the stretch reflex, in which the muscle contracts in reaction to the sudden change of its length and is no better prepared for activity. A better way to warm up before exercise is with dynamic stretching, or gentle motions that mimic some of the movements you'll be making (e.g., arm circles before lifting weights), and a light version of the activity itself (e.g., starting a run by walking, then easing into a jog before picking up the pace).

So, if before working out isn't a good time to work on your flexibility, when is? Two answers: first, after a workout, when your muscles are warm. This can be achieved with static stretching or the alternative described below. For static stretching, target the areas of your body where you're tightest, ease into stretches only to the point of slight tension, keep breathing, increase the length of a stretch only as doing so isn't a strain, and hold each stretch for a minute.

Those short stretching sessions will help to preserve your flexibility. Improving it takes a little more time but is well worth the investment. Two or three fifteen-to-twenty-minute stretching sessions a week will lengthen your muscles, thereby increasing your range of motion and quality of movements. You'll be able to do more regular activities without hurting yourself, including picking up dollar bills from the sidewalk.

If you have the time, doing a longer stretching session after activity is a great time. A stand-alone stretching session has the added benefit of being another time of day when you can discon- nect and focus on yourself. Once you establish a stretching routine, it can take on a meditative or at least calming quality.

Now, about that alternative stretching method. It's called active isolated stretching, or rope stretching. It's based on the premise that muscles work in opposing pairs (quads and hamstrings, biceps and triceps, etc.). To most effectively stretch one of the muscles in the pair, the theory goes, contract its opposite. So to stretch your hamstrings, contract your quads while raising your straight leg from the ground. This allows the hamstrings to relax and gradually lengthen, in contrast to being forced through a range of motion that can cause the stretch reflex to kick in.

Active isolated stretching combines elements of static and dynamic stretching. For each muscle you're stretching, you do ten or so stretches, pausing only at the very end of the stretch, with each stretch lasting only a few seconds. For most of the stretches, you use a rope or towel to assist at the end of the stretch for just a little bit more range of motion. Exhale during the stretching part, inhale while returning to the start position. You can do a whole-body active isolated stretching in less than twenty minutes. You'll feel noticeably better immediately after each one, and measurably more flexible after six weeks of regular sessions.

Good posture also helps your flexibility, because it keeps your muscles in their proper position and length rather than strained and constricted.

#55: Perform Self-Massage

Who doesn't love a massage? While there's nothing quite like an hour under the hands of a skilled therapist, you can produce much of the good of a professional massage on your own with the right self-massage tools.

One big reason you feel so good after a massage is that you've experienced myofascial release. "Myofascial" refers to fascia, the connective tissue that surrounds your muscles and other body parts and allows for movement. This internal webbing can easily stiffen, for reasons such as repetitive motions, inactivity, and improper posture. When your fascia is tight, your mobility, or ability to move freely and easily, is limited.

Many people who feel constricted in their movements think about stretching. As we saw in the previous item, regular stretching is important to maintain or even increase your flexibility. But mobility is equally important to feeling good and performing daily activities without strain. An analogy that Daniel Frey, DPT, uses is Silly Putty. (We met Frey in item #44 about proper workstation ergonomics.) When you first remove Silly Putty from its container, it doesn't have much give. But as you rub it around in your hands, it warms and softens, and can be stretched much farther without breaking. That process, Frey says, is analogous to the increase in mobility you can gain from myofascial release.

One of the best ways to perform self-massage is with a foam roller. The basic motion on a foam roller is to place a body part on it with noticeable, but not painful, pressure, and then roll back and forth for thirty to sixty seconds. Foam rollers are easy to use on the front and back of your legs as well as your upper and lower back.

The classic foam roller is a firm log about six inches in diameter and three feet long, made of polyethylene foam or EVA.

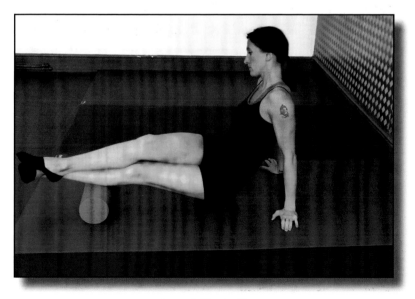

Image via Creative Commons

Manufacturers often color-code their rollers based on firmness, with white usually the softest and black the firmest. Over time, foam rollers can lose their firmness and, therefore, their effectiveness. There are many variations on the basic model, including shorter, hollow rollers with raised areas for extra pressure.

Depending on the body part you're working on, different tools might be called for. Self-massage sticks—the best known is, appropriately, The Stick—are smaller than foam rollers and easy to use on your legs. They're harder to use on your upper body while staying loose and relaxed. Some deeper muscles, such as your glutes and where your hamstrings attach to your pelvis, are difficult to target with larger rolling tools. Gently lowering the area onto a small, firm ball—such as a tennis ball or lacrosse ball—and then rolling around is more effective in these cases.

Self-massage tools can also target trigger points, which are areas in muscles where knots have developed over time. It's possible to have excellent range of motion but still have trigger points that create pain and tightness. Trigger points start as microtears that become chronic through a tear-and-repair repetitive cycle, leading to increased tension in the affected muscle. When working on a trigger point, repeated shorter bouts are better than one longer bout. This approach is similar to what massage therapists do—work on an area to increase blood flow, work elsewhere for a few minutes, then return to the trigger point.

Performing self-massage at least a few times a week, for five to ten minutes at a time, will have a profound impact on your mobility. Myofascial release is safe to do before or after exercise but is effective no matter when you do it. A short session soon before going to bed is a great way to finish the day.

#56: Take a Yoga Class

Or two or three or four, for that matter.

Yoga is rightfully seen by many people as a cornerstone of their health. They value how it builds strength, flexibility, mobility, and balance; encourages mind-body awareness; improves posture, breathing, and mindfulness; and relieves stress.

Those benefits are all available in a good yoga class. I'm recommending you take one or more for a more specific reason: to perform a functional screening of your body.

An all-around yoga class will include a variety of poses—balancing, strengthening, standing, opening, bending, twisting, and more. There will also be gentle restorative poses, probably at the end of the class. It's likely that you'll find some types more challenging than others. That discovery can highlight key things you can do to better your body.

For example, say you find forward bending poses such as Downward Dog to be particularly challenging. This probably means your backside—hamstrings, glutes, lower back, thoracic spine—is too tight and that you should concentrate on improving flexibility in these areas. Maybe you'll find chest opening poses like Camel the most difficult. This probably means your front body is constricted and that you'll benefit from better postural habits. Or maybe strengthening poses like Warrior are the trickiest, indicating, among other things, that you'd benefit from greater hip and glute strength.

You might also find that one side of your body can perform poses better than the other. Differences in how you do a standing pose like Tree reveal strength and balance discrepancies that can cause poor posture, chronic strain on one side of the body, and more. Even something as seemingly simple as Corpse Pose, which looks more or less like lying on your back, can be revelatory, if you find you're unable to relax your mind long enough to just concentrate on your breathing.

#57: Do Cat-Cow Yoga Pose

This yoga posture is a combination of two poses, Marjaryasana (Cat pose) and Bitilasana (Cow pose). It's a gentle vinyasa, or breath-synchronized movement, that almost everyone can easily do. Cat-Cow should be mandatory in offices and anywhere else where people sit most of the day.

That's because Cat-Cow provides immediate relief for much of the tightness that comes from sitting. During the Cat section, your spine will lengthen, your lower back will stretch, and blood flow to the discs between your vertebrae will increase. During the Cow section, your chest will open up, and your head and neck will get a needed elongation. The rhythmic breathing throughout will oxygenate your internal organs.

To do Cat-Cow, start in a neutral position on your hands and knees, with your back flat, your wrists under your shoulders, your knees under your hips, your fingers pointing forward, and your head held gently while you look down.

Start with Cow pose. Inhale as you slowly drop your stomach toward the ground. Lift your chin and chest, and move your ears away from your shoulders. Look up toward the ceiling. Move into Cow pose very gently so as not to strain your lower back.

Then move into Cat pose. Exhale slowly but forcefully as you round your back. Draw your belly button toward your spine and visualize moving the outside of your hips up. Tuck your chin toward your chest without forcing the movement. Try to keep your weight evenly distributed instead of having your shoulders bear the bulk of it.

Return to Cow pose, and move smoothly and continuously between the two poses for ten breaths. Each time, gently stretch your lower back a little more than the previous pose. You'll feel better after just one minute of doing Cat-Cow.

#58: Reset Your Shoulders

Even with diligence about posture and good workstation ergonomics, you might often find yourself slumped forward, either in front of a computer or over a phone. Help your shoulders and neck return to a neutral position, and open up your chest by doing wall slides a few times each work day.

Stand with your back against a wall. Visualize dropping your shoulder blades. Your heels, butt, and head should be touching the wall. While keeping your elbows and the backs of your arms and hands pressed against the wall, raise your arms to a 90-degree angle. If you're unable to keep your hands against the wall in this position, keep your elbows in the same position, and move your hands out a little until they can comfortably rest against the wall.

Slowly but deeply inhale as you slide your arms up and slightly out. By the top of the position, your arms will be straight in a V-shape. Exhale slowly but deeply as you return your arms to the start position. Your head, butt, and feet should remain against the wall throughout. Do ten slides.

If you don't have access to a clear wall, do a variation in a doorway. Stand facing the doorway and place your arms at a 90-degree angle in the doorway, so that your palms are against the surface. Inhale slowly but deeply as you straighten your arms to slide them up. Exhale slowly but deeply as you bring them back to the start position. Maintain good posture throughout, with your head, shoulders, hips, and feet aligned. Do ten slides.

#59: Strengthen Your Neck

The average adult human head weighs ten or eleven pounds. That's a heavy piece of equipment to have perched atop your neck. And when, as is common, your head gets out of position, the rest of your body tends to follow. The result is poor posture and chronic low-grade aches and pains, especially in the neck, shoulders, and upper back.

The most common example of a misaligned head is what's known as forward head, in which your chin is thrust out and your ears, rather than being positioned over your shoulders, are in line with your collar bones. This phenomenon is rife among people who spend a lot of time in front of a computer screen.

It's a good idea, of course, to regularly check your posture, to see if your head, shoulders, hips, and feet are lined up with one another.

But you can greatly increase your chances of maintaining good head posture by doing a simple exercise that strengthens the front of your neck. When those muscles are strong, you can more naturally hold your head erect and in a neutral position.

To do the exercise, all you need is a wall and a small ball with some give, such as a light, hand-held ball weight. While standing tall, place the ball between your forehead and the wall. Push with your forehead to press the ball against the wall. Hold for three seconds, then relax, but maintain enough pressure to keep the ball against the wall. Do ten repetitions, ideally a few times a day on workdays. You should feel an almost immediate repositioning of your head. After two to three weeks, you'll probably notice less discomfort and tightness in your neck and shoulders.

#60: Reset Your Neck

Even after the benefits of the above neck-strengthening exercise kick in, it's easy for your neck muscles to get tight and your head to be out of alignment. Reset your head's position with the following series of neck stretches. Do them all slowly and gently; if your neck and shoulder muscles are under chronic strain, one too-quick move can cause a spasm that might affect you for days.

Start with short sweeps. Stand with your knees slightly bent and your hands on your knees. Drop your head slightly, with your chin tucked toward your chest. Leading with your chin, slowly sweep your head from one side to the other like a pendulum. Begin with a small sweep, and gradually increase the distance over ten sweeps to no farther than your chin coming to shoulder level.

Next, stretch the back of your neck. Stand tall, with your head positioned over your shoulders. Place one hand on your chin and the other on the crown of your head. Exhale as you use your front neck muscles to draw your chin toward your chest. Use your hands only to guide the motion; don't pull your head down. Inhale as you return your head to the starting position. Do ten repetitions.

The last two stretches are for the side neck muscles. Stand tall with your head aligned with your shoulders. Place your right hand over the top of your head so that its fingers are pointing toward your left ear. Exhale as you use the muscles on the right side of your neck to move your head down toward your right shoulder. Don't pull with your hand; use it to slightly increase the stretch at the end of the movement. Inhale as you return your head to the start position. Do ten repetitions on each side.

Return to standing tall with your head positioned over your shoulders. Place your right hand under but not touching your chin. Place your left hand almost in touch with the back of your head. Exhale as you use the muscles of the right side of your neck to turn your head to look toward your right shoulder. Keep your hands hovering in place until you've almost completed the motion, then place them on your head and use them to gently increase the stretch. Inhale as you remove your hands from your head and return your head to the start position. Do ten repetitions on each side.

This quick series will provide significant relief to tired muscles while giving you greater awareness of your head position. Do it two or more times per day during work hours. It's also an easy way to feel better when you're trapped in place during a long plane flight.

#61: Do Bone-Building Activities

The goal here isn't near-immediate improvement, like you can get from muscle-building activities like weight lifting. Instead, it's forestalling an otherwise near-inevitable occurrence—decreased bone density and the frailty that accompanies its advanced form, osteoporosis.

This is oversimplifying, but bone tissue responds to stress in the same basic way that other body parts do: it's temporarily compromised, then, if given adequate recovery, rebuilds stronger in anticipation of encountering the stress again. For muscles, this means becoming bigger to be better able to lift weight; for your circulatory system, this means becoming more efficient at delivering blood; and for your bones, it means becoming denser to better handle impact forces.

The traditional view was that weight-bearing activities were the key to spurring greater bone density. More recent research has shown it's important that the activity have a jarring impact and/or it target bones such as the spine and hips that are common sites of osteoporosis. Running and jumping activities—basketball, tennis, vigorous dancing, jogging—meet these criteria. Strength training that involves the hips and back—think squats, dead lifts, overhead lifts—also works. Low-impact weight-bearing activities such as walking or using an elliptical machine aren't as effective but are better than doing nothing if your current health precludes more high-impact activities.

Note that two popular forms of aerobic exercise, cycling and swimming, don't meet the bone-building criteria. In studies

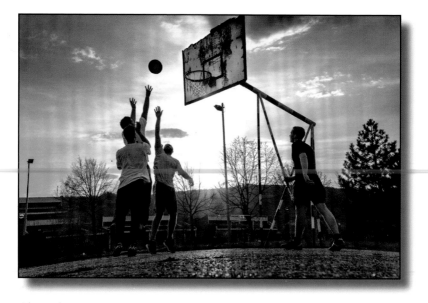

comparing runners, cyclists, and weight lifters, the cyclists tend to have lower bone density. If one of these is your main form of aerobic exercise, you'll want to incorporate twice-weekly strength training.

The bone-building effects from activity accrue slowly over time; studies have found increases of 1 percent or less per year in bone density. This doesn't mean they're insignificant. Without the right activities, adults past the age of thirty can lose anywhere from a fraction of a percent to 2 or more percent of bone density per year. Left unaddressed, these losses accumulate to significant effect over the course of just a decade, for both women and men. The right activities can stave off those declines, leading to a lower risk of fracture, better posture, more independence, and, therefore, greater quality of life.

#62: Improve Your Balance

Put this book down—but only for a short while!—and try an experiment.

From a standing position, lift one foot off the ground so that it's parallel with the other knee. Then close your eyes.

How'd that go for you? If you're like most people, as soon as you shut your eyes you began to wobble. You may have even started to fall over.

What that exercise tests is your proprioception, or your sense of spatial orientation. Proprioceptors are sensors in your muscles and tendons that constantly assess the movement and orientation of your body in relation to the surrounding environment. Proprioceptors

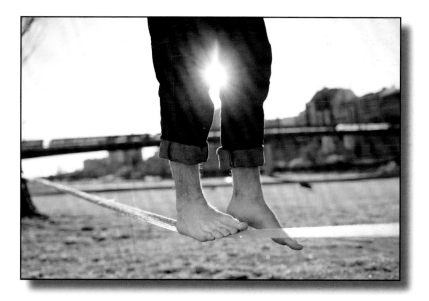

help you quickly catch yourself and stay on your feet when you do something like unexpectedly step on a wet floor or an unseen object. Closing your eyes in the above balance test makes you rely solely on your proprioceptors (and makes you realize how, without your thinking about it, vision plays a key role in balance).

Improving your proprioception will help you to avoid falls, ankle sprains, and other consequences of what you might ascribe to clumsiness. You'll also be better able to navigate tricky terrain and poorly lit environments.

A simple way to do so is repeat the above balance exercise twice a day on each foot. Start by balancing on each foot for a minute at a time, with your eyes open. When that's no longer challenging, do it with your eyes shut. A convenient time to do two minutes of balance exercises twice a day is when you brush your teeth in the morning and evening.

A nice thing about balance exercises is that your central nervous system learns quickly. Within a week you should start to notice marked improvement.

#63: Do Planks

Adequate strength in your midsection is essential to maintaining good posture. Without good core stability, you're more likely to sit, stand, and move in ways that will throw your body out of alignment, setting you up for chronic low-grade strains and discomfort from your neck all the way down to your feet.

Planks are a simple way to build basic core strength. The three variations described below are quick, convenient, and effective

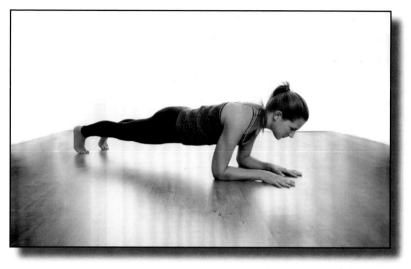

Image via Creative Commons

do-anywhere exercises. For each, stay in the position only as long as you can maintain the proper form. Over time, work up to holding each for one minute. Devoting a few minutes most days to doing planks will give you a stable base for daily activities.

Start with a prone plank. Lie on the ground flat on your stomach. Place your forearms flat on the ground with your elbows under your shoulders. Lift your body off of the ground and make a straight line through your ankles, knees, hips, shoulders, and head. Focus on keeping your stomach and glutes tight. Stop if your hips drop or lift up, or if your stomach sags.

Next, turn over and do a supine plank. Lie on the ground flat on your back. Place your forearms flat on the ground with your elbows under your shoulders. Use your glutes and lower back muscles to raise yourself so that your elbows and heels are in touch with the ground. Keep a straight line through your ankles, knees, hips, shoulders, and head. Don't thrust your hips higher than the rest of your body. Stop if your hips sag or you start to shake.

Finally, do side planks. Lie on one side with your top leg slightly in front of your bottom. Place the forearm on the down side against the ground and under your shoulder. Raise your hips off the ground, balancing on your feet and arm. Maintain a straight line along your feet, hips, spine, and head. Be careful not to let your hips sag toward the ground. Repeat on your other side.

#64: Do Push-Ups

Adequate upper-body strength is crucial for getting through daily activities without injury and frustration. Because few of us do work that requires and therefore builds upper-body strength, we need to take time to nurture it.

Push-ups are to upper-body strength as planks are to core strength. They're quick, convenient, and effective; and for people who just need the basic benefits, they're good enough. Done properly, push-ups will strengthen your shoulders, chest, triceps, abs, and more, and improve your posture. They're a great example of how simple exercises build functional fitness, the sort that is broadly applicable to many activities rather than specific to one sport and muscle group.

To do a basic push-up, place your hands on the ground under your shoulders, with your arms straight. With your weight balanced evenly between your hands and toes, align your body from your ankles through your hips on up to your shoulders. Slightly contract your abs and back leg muscles to help you maintain this straight position. Keep your neck relaxed and your head in line with the rest of your body.

Inhale as you lower your chest to the ground. Focus on keeping your back flat and your head aligned with your shoulders. Don't let your hips sag or point up. Keep your elbows close to your torso. Exhale to return to the start position, always focusing on keeping your body aligned.

Do only as many as you can with proper form. A few good push-ups done correctly are better than three times as many with bad mechanics. Don't try to increase the number you do every time. As your strength increases and you become more familiar with holding the proper form, you'll naturally be able to start doing more. If you can properly do twenty to twenty-five push-ups at a time and want to continue progressing, increase your volume of push-ups by adding one or more additional push-up sessions during

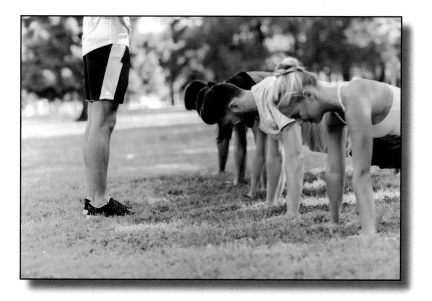

the day rather than doing more all in one session. Trying to do too many at once can overload your lower back.

#65: Strengthen Your Grip

Research has found grip strength to be an indicator of overall muscular strength and endurance. A good grip is necessary if you have the laudable goal of lifting weights to strength other parts of your body. And good grip strength makes daily activities such as carrying shopping bags or luggage and opening jars easier.

You've no doubt seen a hand gripper, the two-handled device built for the sole purpose of strengthening your grip. A few sessions per day of squeezing it with each hand for twenty to thirty seconds at a time will give you more than enough grip strength for daily life.

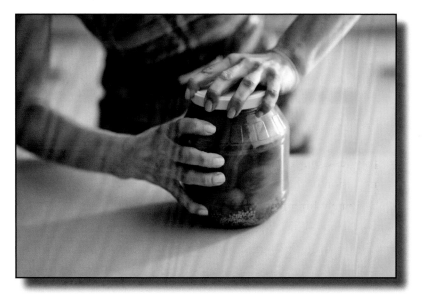

You can also build that aspect of grip strength, called crush grip, by performing the same action with a stress ball or a soft material such as a washcloth or newspaper wadded up into a ball.

A convenient way to build support grip strength, which is what you use when carrying something, is to do a farmer's carry. Wrap each hand around a dumbbell or kettlebell and walk around a room for a minute. A weighted watering can also works here. The final type of grip strength is called pinch grip, which you use to grab and hold something between your thumb and fingers. Use the device you carried in the farmer's carry, but stand in place while holding it with a pinch grip for up to one minute per hand.

#66: Lift with Your Legs

Here's a case where the conventional wisdom is both correct and often unheeded.

The biggest, strongest muscles in your body are between your butt and knees. Yet many people lift items on the ground by bending over the item and pulling up with their arms while keeping their legs mostly or entirely straight. Lifting like this removes the legs from the equation and places most of the load on your lower back and spine. Doing so is not only ineffective but also dangerous, with compression of the spinal discs and/or lower back pain possible.

To safely lift a heavy object off the ground, stand in front of it with your feet shoulder-width apart, with one foot a little in front of the other. Squat in front of the object by bending your hips and knees while keeping your back straight and your shoulders unhunched.

This next step is crucial: grasp the item and begin ever so slightly to come up. At this time, make a realistic assessment of whether you can lift the object. We all have our limits; it's better to underestimate your strength and ask for help than find out the object is too heavy as you hurt yourself.

If you determine you can safely lift it, rise slowly by pushing up with your legs. Protect your back by keeping it straight and not turning. Increase the stability of your lift by keeping the object close to your body at stomach level. Once you're erect, maintain a straight back. Initiate changes in direction with your feet and hips, not your upper body.

If you have a history of back problems, or if you've been idle for a while, such as first thing in the morning, use the above technique even when lifting lighter items.

#67: Use Over-the-Counter Painkillers Sparingly

The usual reason given for not mindlessly downing ibuprofen and other nonprescription painkillers is your internal health. Use of these popular drugs has been linked to two types of kidney problems. One, acute renal failure, is a relatively rare emergency situation caused by short-term use, most often in certain vulnerable populations. The second type of kidney problem is long-term, brought on by regular use of these drugs over years. These problems occur because the drugs are excreted through the kidneys rather than broken down by the liver or passed through your digestive tract.

Those are good reasons to take the drugs only as prescribed. Here's another: pain is your body's signal that something is wrong. Regularly masking that pain treats the symptoms but not the underlying cause.

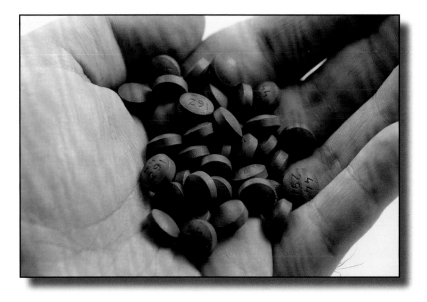

There's always a balance between getting some relief from pain and making good use of what your body is trying to tell you. Let's say you wake in the middle of the night with a throbbing jaw. You get up, gobble a handful of ibuprofen, and eventually get back to sleep. You might wake the next morning and find the issue has resolved itself. Alternatively, you might wake and again feel the throbbing. In this case, you keep taking painkillers, but when the drugs wear off, the throbbing is worse, so you take more painkillers. After a week of this you can't take it anymore, see a dentist, learn you have an abscessed tooth, and get the proper treatment.

Even more typical is some people's practice of taking OTC pain-killers for chronic low-grade issues, such as sciatic pain or shoulder stiffness. In these cases, you're putting yourself at risk for long-term kidney damage while ignoring what could be a fixable problem with your body. Your sciatic pain might stem from too much sitting and a weak backside. Your shoulder strain might stem from poor posture at work and too much time bent over your phone. In the absence of painkillers, you can better hear your body's messages and make a plan to address the underlying issue.

CHAPTER 4

16 Things to Do to Improve Your Internal Health and Fitness

The tips in this chapter are mostly about diet, with a few having to do with other aspects of keeping your insides well-functioning.

#68: Stay Properly Hydrated

Proper hydration is essential to health. It's unlikely you'll get severely dehydrated, which carries severe consequences, in day-to-day life, even if you exercise a lot. Chronic mild to moderate dehydration, however, is still worth avoiding, as it can cause headaches, low energy, dry skin, constipation, dizziness, and other disruptive symptoms.

Note that I said "proper hydration." That's not the same as obsessive hydration. Your body loses water through sweating and other processes, and it can handle those losses in the short term without your having to immediately replace them. Much of the impetus for people to tote water or sport drinks everywhere comes from manufacturers of those products. When you drink more than your body needs, your urine output increases; depending on what you're drinking, you might be literally pissing away your money.

What is proper hydration? It's an amount that strikes the balance between your not being thirsty and not running off to the bathroom every hour.

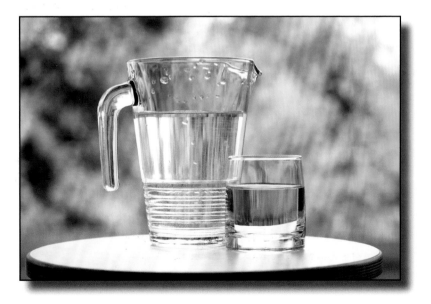

You may have heard that you should drink eight glasses of water a day. This advice doesn't take two facts into account. First, people of different sizes and activity levels have different fluid needs. Second, all fluids count toward meeting your hydration needs. So does food—some fruits and vegetables are primarily water. Fruit juice, milk, tea, beer, coffee, and other liquids all help to keep you hydrated.

Caffeinated and alcoholic beverages have traditionally been considered diuretic, meaning that they dehydrate you by inducing urination. The expert consensus now is that these drinks count toward meeting your fluid needs. They can increase your urine output in the short term, but then a compensatory mechanism results in your holding on to more water over the ensuing twenty-four hours.

Most of the time, you can stay adequately hydrated by listening to your body; if you're thirsty, drink something. Keep fluids you like nearby so that you're more likely to sip when you feel the urge. In warm weather, when you're more likely to get dehydrated, make more of an effort to gauge your thirst. When it's hot, monitor the color of your urine. If you're properly hydrated, it should be a pale yellow. If it turns darker, drink more.

#69: Go Easy on the Sport Drinks

As someone who sweats heavily and regularly does two-hour runs drinking water or nothing, I'm here to tell you that most people don't need sport drinks most of the time.

One of the first sport drinks, Gatorade, was created to help University of Florida football players survive hours-long practices under a broiling sun. Gatorade and similar drinks have been shown to improve performance in high-intensity endurance events such as marathons and long bicycle races. The performance boost comes primarily because the carbohydrates in the drink are quickly used by working muscles. This prolongs the body's stores of preserved carbo-hydrate, glycogen, which is muscles' preferred source of fuel during aerobic activity.

It takes a lot of work to significantly draw down your glycogen stores, like running fifteen to twenty miles at a good clip. At lower intensities, such as a day-long hike, a greater percentage of your energy comes from burning fat, which the body has more than enough of for such purposes, even in the leanest among us. There

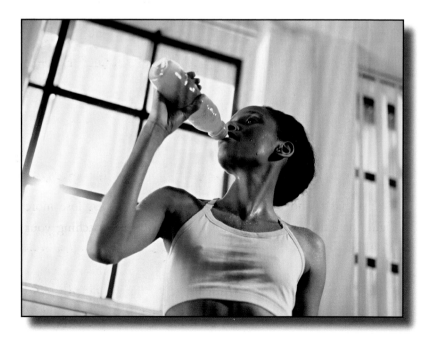

is no risk of running low on glycogen—and therefore no need of carbohydrate supplementation—during the sorts of workouts most people do.

Sport drinks are also said to be necessary to replace the fluids and electrolytes (sodium, potassium, etc.) lost in sweat. Short-term light to moderate dehydration, such as you might experience after an hour of using an elliptical machine or mowing the lawn, is normal and not harmful. You're not putting yourself at risk if you don't immediately replace your fluid losses. Water and a normal healthy diet will replenish your fluid and electrolyte losses.

A one-quart bottle of a typical sport drink contains about 200 calories, all of which come from simple sugars, but no significant nutrients. If you're watching your weight, that quart bottle adds to your calorie count without meeting basic nutrition needs.

These drinks can be refreshing when you're really dehydrated. By spurring more drinking, the sodium in them can help you to rehydrate more quickly. But you shouldn't consider them necessary or even helpful for normal life, which includes regular moderate exercise.

#70: Read Food Labels

Research has found that dieters who read food labels lose more weight than those who don't. Even if you're not watching your weight, learning how to make sense of food labels can improve your health.

I like to start with the ingredient list. It shows ingredients in descending order by weight, so the first few you see are the main things you'll consume. Decide if they're what you really want from this item. For example, if you were to make pasta sauce at home, would one of the main ingredients be sugar? Probably not. But it is in some bottled sauces. (See the following item for more on added sugar.)

The other key things to look for are preservatives, which enable a food to be packaged, shipped a long distance, and sit on a shelf for a long time; and additives, which enhance flavor and/or appearance. They're not all going to give you cancer after one serving, but for a balanced diet, lean more toward avoiding them than eating them. I often tell myself I should avoid a product if I can't pronounce a sizable number of its ingredients.

The label will detail how much of the food's calories are from fat. Focus on the amounts of saturated fat and trans fat. A good goal is to get less than 10 percent of your calories from saturated fat, which raises your cholesterol level. This doesn't mean that every food you

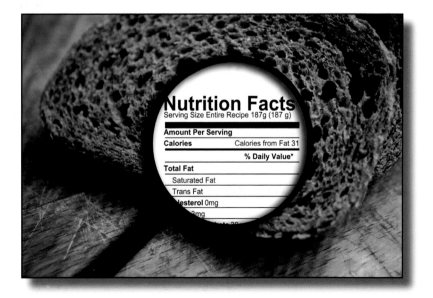

buy should get less than 10 percent of its calories from saturated fat, given that many foods have none. On balance, however, try to buy ones that are low in saturated fat. As much as possible, avoid foods with trans fat, which not only raises your LDL ("bad") cholesterol, but also lowers your HDL ("good") cholesterol, increasing your risk for heart disease. Try not to consume more than two grams of trans fat per day.

If you're concerned about your weight, carefully read the information at the top about the number of calories per serving. In recent years, listed serving sizes have become more in line with reality—no more listing half an English muffin as a serving—so it's easier to get a good idea of the item's caloric value. Nonetheless, compare the listed serving size to how you eat the food to more accurately determine if it's a good choice for you. A bag of potato chips, for example, might show that a serving of ten chips contains fifty-six calories. If that's an amount you can be satisfied with, the pleasure the chips bring could be worth the relatively modest calorie count. If, however, you know you're going to wind up eating forty chips, then they're moving toward not helping you meet your goals.

#71: Beware of Added Sugar

Starting in 2018, reading food labels will be even more useful. In addition to the current requirement to list total sugars, labels will have to show how much added sugar a product has.

This will be useful information, because, as we saw above, sugar is added to many packaged foods that you might not suspect contain it—salad dressings, fruit drinks, yogurt, ketchup, cole slaw, granola, energy bars, instant oatmeal, and on and on. These unexpected sources of sugar make it easy to exceed the World Health Organization's recommendation to consume no more than six teaspoons of added sugar per day.

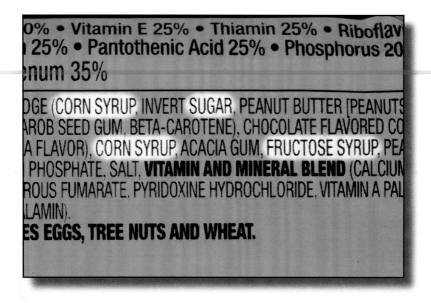

The revised food labels will have a more generous recommendation of 50 grams, or about twelve teaspoons. If you visualize twelve teaspoons, it might seem like a lot. But consider that a small container of flavored yogurt might contain five teaspoons. One ounce of ketchup might contain one and a half teaspoons. And that doesn't take into account added sugar you consume from more obvious sources, such as jelly, baked goods, and soft drinks.

Added sugar plays a big role in many people's struggle with their weight. It's also linked to an increased risk for conditions like type 2 diabetes and heart disease.

Food is one of life's great pleasures. Most experts say consuming added sugar in moderation can fit into a healthful diet. The point here is to be mindful of not getting too much from unsuspected sources so that, if you choose, you can have your cake and eat it, too.

#72: Choose Food Over Supplements

If you're supposed to eat lots of fruits and vegetables for their nutrients, then why not just take a pill that delivers those nutrients? With a few exceptions—see the following item, for example—opting for supplements instead of food is a bad idea.

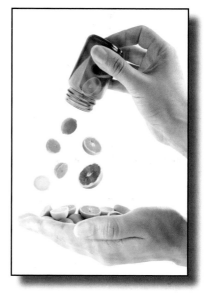

Foods are more than the sum of their parts; broccoli isn't just a delivery system for vitamin A, nor is a banana merely a potassium pill with a peel. They contain other beneficial compounds beyond vitamins and minerals, such as flavonoids and fiber. In addition, it's believed the various compounds in food work together to produce their benefits. Humans evolved eating complex foods; we currently don't know how to better that process with pills.

Also, the pills-over-food mindset can make it more likely that you'll disregard the quality of your diet. You might think, "I took my daily multivitamin, so why not have pie for breakfast?" Replacing nutrient-dense foods with those of lesser quality will probably mean eating more processed foods, saturated fat, and other things that are known to increase your risk of common lifestyle diseases.

It's also easier to get too much of a nutrient from supplements. Ours is a more-is-better society, and it might seem logical that if a certain amount of a vitamin is good, then three times as much is three times as good. Vitamin overdoses are rare from food but can occur with supplements. One of the most commonly taken supplements, vitamin C, can cause problems such as diarrhea and nausea when taken in excess.

#73: Watch Your Vitamin D Status in the Winter

Vitamin D plays many roles in the body, including absorbing calcium and building bone. Those two functions are why milk is often fortified with vitamin D.

There's growing expert consensus that vitamin D is vital to proper immune system function, and that the challenge to maintaining a sufficient vitamin D level in the winter causes people to have more colds and flus at that time of the year.

What's the challenge? Sunlight, or, more accurately, lack of sunlight. Vitamin D is primarily obtained through the ultraviolet B rays of the sun. Between latitudes of 30 degrees north and 60 degrees north—from Houston to just south of Anchorage, Alaska—it takes only fifteen minutes of midday sun to provide about 80 percent of the recommended daily allowance.

In the winter, not only is there far less sunlight, but what sunlight there is transmits negligible amounts of ultraviolet B rays to the skin. In addition, many people are indoors for large chunks of the scant daylight time. Because it's nearly impossible to get as much vitamin D from food as is easily obtained from the sun, vitamin D levels can plummet in the winter.

Experts in the topic distinguish between vitamin D deficiency and vitamin D sufficiency. Deficiency occurs at blood levels below 25 nmol/liter; in that state, your immunity is likely to be

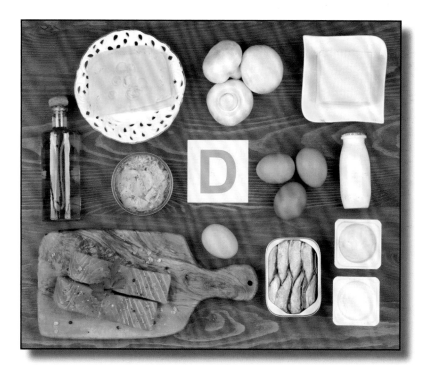

compromised. Sufficiency has usually been tagged at 50 nmol/liter; here, your immune system is reasonably strong. Studies have found large percentages of people fall below that level in the winter.

One leading researcher has found that people who maintain a level of 75 nmol/liter in the winter get fewer colds and flus and show evidence of stronger immune function. Reaching this level means taking in about 1,000 international units (IU) of vitamin D per day. During the winter, the sun will contribute almost nothing to hitting that goal. Doing so through diet is almost impossible, even with fortified foods. For example, a six-ounce salmon steak, which is one of the leading dietary sources of vitamin D, contains about 425 IUs. A large boiled egg, another top source of vitamin D, has about 260 IUs. Hope you're hungry!

These facts support taking a daily 1,000 IU vitamin D supplement in the winter. Look for those packaged as vitamin D3.

#74: Eat Home-Cooked Meals

Research has found that people who usually cook dinner at home have diets that are lower in fat and sugar than the diets of people who seldom eat home-cooked dinners. In addition, even among those not trying to lose weight, people who regularly eat home-cooked dinners consume fewer calories per day than infrequent cooks.

In one study, people who cooked dinner six to seven times a week (48 percent of the participants) consumed 2,164 calories, 81 grams of fat, and 119 grams of sugar in a typical day. Those who cooked dinner once or zero times per week (8 percent of the participants) consumed 2,301 calories, 84 grams of fat, and 135 grams of sugar in a typical day.

Regular home-cooked meals have also been found to benefit kids. In one review of studies on the matter, researchers found that children from families who eat a lot of meals together at home have better diets and lower body mass index than those from families who eat out frequently.

Children who frequently eat at home with their families eat more fruit, vegetables, fiber, and calcium- and vitamin-rich foods. The more a child's family eats out, the greater the amount of less nutritious food and drinks, such as soft drinks, he or she consumes.

#75: Keep a Well-Stocked Cupboard

Remember the first tip in this book? It was about choice architecture, or setting up your life so that it's easier to make good choices. The state of your pantry is an excellent example of the importance of good choice architecture.

Consider a scenario in which you get home from work late and have been go-go-go since the morning. You're tired, stressed, mentally drained, and hungry. What's for dinner?

As we saw in the previous item, meals prepared at home tend to be lower in fat and calories than those from restaurants. That's especially the case in I'm-famished-and-there's-nothing-to-eat-here situations, when you're more likely to opt for fast food, a deli sandwich, pizza delivery, and the like. A healthful home-cooked meal will not only be better for your waistline and cholesterol level, but will probably leave you feeling better than ending your stressful day with a heap of fried food.

But to do the right thing in this situation, you need to be prepared for its inevitability. (After all, the odds are low you're going to head to the grocery store, then come back home and start cooking.) With a few staples always on hand, it's easy to quickly assemble a satisfying, nutritious meal. What those staples are will vary from person to person, depending on your typical diet. For some, it will be pasta and frozen vegetables, while others might pull a chicken breast from the freezer or mix canned beans with rice for an impromptu burrito. The key is to have everything you need—cooking oil, grains, protein, vegetables—within reach to easily make one of your go-to workday meals.

If you struggle to eat well in the morning, this same approach applies to breakfast. Again, the particulars will vary by

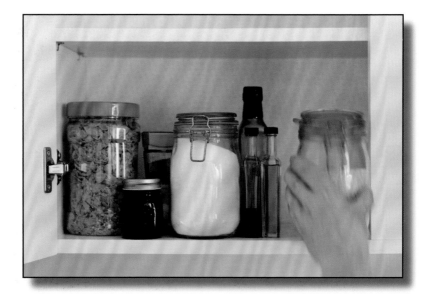

individual—quick oats and dried fruit for some, eggs or cereal and yogurt for others. But the underlying premise of making it easy to do the right thing is universal.

#76: Rinse Produce

In Chapter 1, we saw a strong argument for buying organic versions of some common fruits and vegetables as a way to avoid pesticide residue. (See item #14.) A separate step in food safety is to rinse almost all produce, whether grown organically or conventionally, to remove harmful bacteria.

Consider: there are an estimated seventy-six million cases of foodborne illness in the United States each year. Many of the bacteria that cause foodborne illness, such as *E. coli* and *Salmonella*,

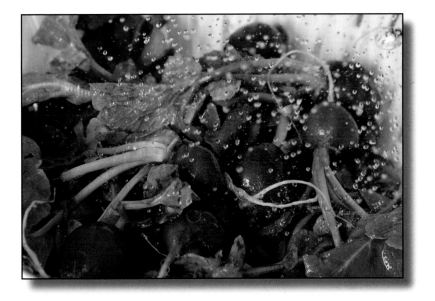

can be found on produce. Fortunately, rinsing produce with potable water removes nearly all bacteria.

Research has found that a thorough rinse with water that's safe to drink does as good a job or better than commercial food sprays in removing bacteria. If you're not a fan of your local tap water, filter it before rinsing with it, or use distilled water.

The need to rinse produce isn't affected by how lovingly something is grown, be it in your garden or by a local farmer. There's always the possibility that the food has been handled by someone with potentially dangerous bacteria on their hands. Similarly, the soil in which the food was grown could contain contaminants. To be safe, wash it. The exceptions are packaged produce labeled as "washed" or "ready to eat." These foods are safe to eat as is.

Speaking of being safe, wash your hands before handling produce to remove the possibility of your being the person who made you sick.

Unprocessed fruits and vegetables are a cornerstone of a good diet. Don't let the simple step of rinsing keep you from eating them daily.

#77: Eat Fermented Foods

Foods such as sauerkraut, kimchi, and yogurt owe their unique taste to fermentation. That's a method of food preparation in which bacteria convert the sugars in the given food into lactic acid. (In beer and some other fermented beverages, yeasts convert the sugar into alcohol.) This natural process has been used by humans for thousands of year as a way to preserve food. As it turns out, fermentation also has health benefits.

The bacteria in fermented foods are considered probiotics, which are live microorganisms in food that confer a benefit to the host (in this case, you). In the case of fermented foods, those benefits are many.

First, in the process of fermentation, foods become more vitamin-potent, and the minerals in them become easier for the body to absorb. In studies, fermented foods have been found to help with some intestinal inflammatory conditions, such as irritable bowel syndrome and ulcerative colitis. Anecdotally, many people value fermented foods for aiding digestion.

Research has also shown probiotics to boost immune system function and to lessen the symptoms of lactose intolerance. In addition, one study found that university students who added kimchi to their diet for a week had lower cholesterol levels at the end of the week, with those who ate the most kimchi experiencing a greater drop than those who ate less.

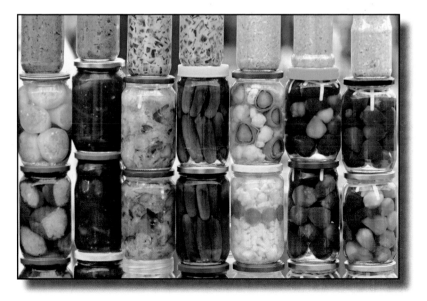

Probiotics are most often touted for improving the state of and diversity of the gut microbiome. The important thing to remember here is that not all bacteria are harmful. The ones associated with fermented foods are thought to carry out beneficial processes, including reducing the number of "bad" bacteria resident in the gut that can cause disease. Probiotics are increasingly recommended for people who are prescribed antibiotics for a medical condition, as a way to lessen antibiotic side effects such as diarrhea.

Be sure you're eating fermented foods that contain probiotics. Many commercially available fermented foods, including sauerkraut and kimchi, have been pasteurized and cooked at high heat, which kills the helpful bacteria. If you're not up for making your own, look for small-batch, locally made versions that haven't been cooked. For dairy products, look on the label for the words "live cultures." These products contain probiotics and are the ones you want.

#78: Swap Spinach for Iceberg Lettuce, and Other Satisfying Salad Substitutions

It's normal to feel virtuous when you eat a typical salad. How could a bunch of raw vegetables not be a healthful choice, regardless of what the rest of your meal looks like? Well . . .

When most people think about improving the nutritional quality of their garden salads, they look to the dressing. And that's always a good idea. Two tablespoons of a typical bottled Thousand Island dressing, for example, gets about 75 percent of its 130 calories from fat, contains 14 percent of the recommended daily intake of sodium, and has three grams of added sugar in the form of high-fructose corn syrup. Its beneficial nutrients are negligible— just 2 percent of a day's need for calcium.

But it's also worth considering what you're putting the dressing on.

One cup of iceberg lettuce, the most common ingredient in a garden-variety garden salad, has ten calories. That low number, and iceberg's ready availability, has long been part of its appeal. But other than being a conveyor of dressing, the lettuce has relatively little to recommend it. A one-cup serving provides 7 percent of your daily vitamin A needs, and much smaller amounts of the other nutrients it contains, such as vitamin C and iron.

Contrast that with the same amount of spinach. It has sven calories, which is a little less than iceberg, but a negligible difference in the grand scheme of things. Many people would say that

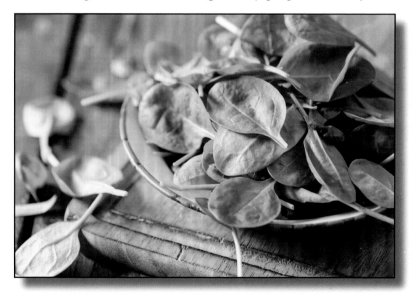

spinach tastes better. That's a matter of taste, but there's no denying that spinach is much more nutritionally dense. For your one cup of greens, you get eight times as much vitamin A as in iceberg, or more than half your daily need. You also get 14 percent of your daily vitamin C needs—almost five times more than in iceberg—and meaningful amounts of iron, dietary fiber, niacin, and zinc.

Similar satisfying substitutions are available with other greens. With just one cup of baby kale in your salad, you'll more than meet your daily needs for vitamins A and C, and get almost 10 percent of your recommended calcium and iron. The same amount of mesclun supplies 30 percent of your vitamin A needs. A cup of romaine, probably the most readily available green at salad bars other than iceberg, contains 81 percent of the vitamin C you need each day.

The point isn't to never eat iceberg. But when you're building your next garden salad, consider it, well, the tip of the iceberg.

#79: When You Eat, Just Eat

You might want to rethink lunching at your desk or watching Netflix during dinner. Research has found that doing things like watching television or reading while eating can lead to eating more calories, both during the meal and later in the day.

Several studies have compared subjects who simply ate and others who dined while doing something else. The findings are consistent: when people engage in other activities while eating, they tend to eat more. When people pay attention to their meals, they tend to better align their consumption with their level of hunger. It can take several minutes for your body to send the "I'm full" signal;

during the interim it's easier to mindlessly overeat if you're staring at a screen or flipping through your phone.

Even if you don't eat too much during your distracted dining, you might later in the day. One review of research on the topic found that people who multitasked at meal time were worse at accurately recalling how much they had eaten at a previous meal, and that this often led to eating more than they otherwise would have at subsequent meals.

The consequences of distracted eating are another good reason to eat with others. Communal meals are well known as a way to build family and social bonds. Taking time to converse slows the pace of a meal, putting the end of the meal closer to the time when your brain updates you on your appetite. Synching your eating with others can also make meals longer. Few people want to be the one with a clean plate when their companion is only halfway through the meal.

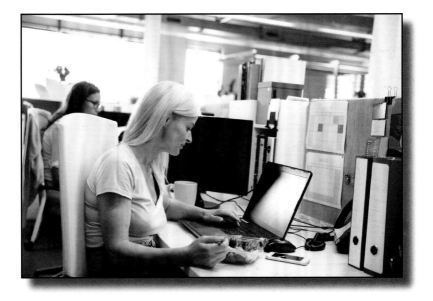

But please, when you eat with others, put your phone away. In addition to being rude, checking your phone while eating puts you back in the distracted-eater category and detracts from some of the meal's social benefits. One study even found that merely the presence of a phone on the table lowered feelings of empathy and connection.

#80: Keep a Food Journal

Writing down everything you eat and drink sounds like the sort of joy-draining task that can drive you to seek comfort in a pint of ice cream. I'm not advocating keeping a food journal for the rest of your life. I am suggesting that keeping one for a week can help you discover patterns that might be hindering your health.

The first thing you can learn is how often and how much you eat. In some studies, people who recorded everything they put in their mouths lost more weight than dieters who didn't keep a food journal. It's likely that realizing they'd have to write down "grabbed handful of M&Ms from office kitchen" kept some people from said grab.

Along the same lines, many studies have found that people tend to underestimate portion size. Thinking to yourself, "I had a few chips while making dinner," is far less revealing than writing "twenty-four potato chips while making dinner." Getting an accurate handle on an average day's consumption can help you see if you need to cut back on frequency and/or portions to be at your desired weight.

Including the situation when you ate can reveal patterns of self-sabotage. Many of us eat in times of stress or boredom, even when we're not hungry. Identifying the "why" that accompanies the "what" can help reduce unnecessary calories and motivate you to come up with better coping strategies in those situations.

A food journal can also help you clarify how you react to certain foods. Are you really lactose- or gluten-intolerant? Keep a journal for one week in which you eat those foods, then for another week when you don't, and make notes of your energy level and digestion. Less dramatically, a simple document of what you ate when and how you felt throughout the day can show things like what size dinner you sleep best after, how much coffee is too much, what type of lunch best energizes you for the afternoon, and so on.

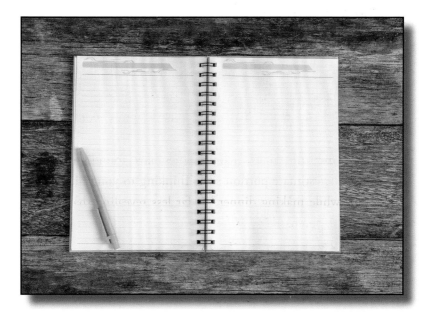

#81: Clean Your House

There are indications that too-clean homes can lead to infants developing allergies and asthma later in life. The theory is that a little exposure to dust and other allergens early on helps to build resistance at later ages.

Let's be honest—"too clean" isn't a phrase most of us would ascribe to our homes. For most of us, a little more cleanliness will likely bring health benefits. Yes, that includes the dust and other allergens that might help infants build immunity. Too much of these substances can lead to respiratory problems.

Kitchen counters and table tops can host potentially harmful bacteria in your home. As we saw earlier in this chapter, there are millions of cases of foodborne illness each year in the United States. A clean kitchen and eating area lowers your risk of transferring bacteria from your hands to food. Another issue associated with

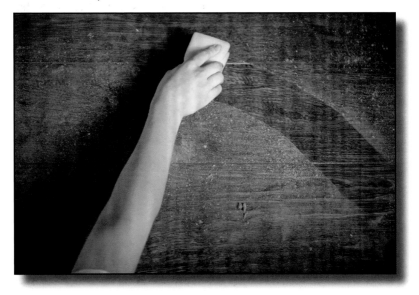

the kitchen, such as mold, can be present anywhere in the house, including bathrooms. Some molds and mold spores can cause cold- or flu-like symptoms, especially to people with weakened immune systems.

#82: Avoid Secondhand Smoke

If you're among the more than 80 percent of Americans who don't smoke, congratulations. As we saw in Chapter 1, not smoking is one of the most important things you can do to be in good health.

Unfortunately, you're still at risk if you're regularly around others who are smoking. Even small amounts are harmful. The American Cancer Society says there's no safe amount of exposure to second-hand smoke. Exposure to secondhand smoke means exposure to nicotine and the same carcinogens that can kill smokers, and the greater your exposure, the greater your risk.

The biggest risk is lung cancer. Several other types of cancer, including throat, brain, breast, and stomach, have been linked to secondhand smoke. Heart and mental health problems are also possible. The risks are even greater for children, who can suffer asthma, bronchitis, and ear infections, among other conditions.

There are two types of secondhand smoke, mainstream (what the smoker exhales) and sidestream (what's produced by the burning end of a cigarette). Of the two, sidestream smoke contains greater concentrations of carcinogens. It also has smaller particles of smoke, meaning that it can more easily enter your lungs and bloodstream. Sidestream smoke is especially worth avoiding.

Smoking is now prohibited in most workplaces and public places such as restaurants and airports. Yet exposure is still possible in public places such as streets and, especially, smoking-designated areas outside bars, shopping centers, and the like. Occupants of multi-unit housing, or guests in hotels that allow smoking in some rooms, can be contaminated as smoke moves through small openings in buildings. Again, no amount of secondhand smoke is safe. When necessary, vote with your wallet to avoid secondhand smoke.

#83: Do Kegel Exercises

If you're a guy and think this tip doesn't apply to you, think again.

Kegels are best known as an exercise prescribed for pregnant women and new mothers. Kegels strengthen the muscles of the pelvic floor. These muscles can weaken during pregnancy and after childbirth, leading to severe discomfort from the womb and bladder not being properly supported.

Weak pelvic floor muscles can also lead to urinary incontinence, which is a strong urge to urinate soon before voiding a large amount of urine. And here's where men come in, because with age they become more susceptible to urinary incontinence, especially if they've had treatment (surgery or radiation therapy) for prostate cancer.

The first step in doing Kegels is to find the right muscles to exercise. A simple way to do so is to stop and start urinating, and to repeat a few times. Pay attention to how deep these muscles are when you contract them. Notice that to most effectively stop your urine, you don't use your stomach or leg muscles. Once you know which muscles to use, don't make a habit of stopping and starting your urine flow, as doing so can lead to a urinary tract infection.

Kegels are simply replicating the contractions you did to stop your urine flow. Ideally, you'll do the exercises when your bladder is empty. Contract your pelvic floor muscles for a count of five, relax for a few seconds, and repeat five times. Do this two to three times a day. Over time, build up to three sets of 10 ten-count repeats per day. When you're first learning Kegels, do them lying down. As you become more familiar with them, you can also do them sitting or standing, at any time during the day. If you're doing them correctly, no one will know what you're up to.

CHAPTER 5

17 Things to Do to Improve Your Mental Health

In this final chapter, we'll look at how to improve your happiness, better your mood, and boost your mental acuity.

#84: Be Physically Active

If the myriad of physical benefits of exercise aren't enough to motivate you to work out regularly, then maybe the mental benefits will do the trick.

By "mental benefits," I don't just mean the well-being that occurs during and after workouts, thanks to the release of endorphins. Nor do I mean only how exercise can lead to improved levels of the mood-boosting neurotransmitters serotonin and norepinephrine. Those relatively short-term benefits are accompanied by changes in the brain that better your cognitive abilities now and in the future.

Studies have found that regular exercisers do better than sedentary people at tests similar to some office work, including the ability to pay attention, memory and making progress on more than one task at a time. Research on school children has found that fitter kids are better learners.

These benefits are likely explained in part by this fact: aerobic exercise such as running and cycling is known to help the brain create new neurons (the type of brain cell often called "gray matter") and blood vessels. These types of workouts may also increase the size of the hippocampus, which is associated with memory and learning, and the midbrain, which is associated with vision and hearing. Quite simply, regular exercise builds a bigger brain.

As long as you keep exercising, those beneficial changes in brain structure and capacity are likely to last into your later years. There's overwhelming evidence that active older people have less brain shrinkage and signs of cognitive decline. In one study with a five-year follow-up period, the people with the most gray matter related to physical activity were half as likely to experience memory decline or get Alzheimer's disease.

It's never too late to start exercising to get the physical benefits. Research has shown that to be true of the mental benefits, as well. Being active is always the smart thing to do.

#85: Stop Multitasking

Let's say you started reading this sentence but then heard your phone ding because you got a text. Even if you glanced over and decided the text didn't warrant putting down the fascinating book you hold in your hand, it's too late. Those couple of seconds were enough to distract you. Now, where were you?

People who constantly multitask pride themselves on their productivity and efficiency. Trouble is, research has consistently shown these people are wrong, and that constantly flitting from one task to another impairs mental functioning.

A big reason multitaskers are mistaken is that they're not really multitaskers. Instead, the way the human brain works means that they're rapidly switching from one task to another. Working in this manner has been shown to result in lower, not higher, productivity, because some of the brain's finite resources are devoted to the act of switching between tasks. And because the brain experiences switching between tasks as an interruption, multitasking also fails on the efficiency front. Studies have shown that interruptions as brief as two to three seconds cause people to perform significantly worse compared to performing the same task without interruptions.

Multitasking's always-on mode can lead to a higher heart rate and increased levels of the stress hormone cortisol. These two physical phenomena, combined with the lower productivity and efficiency of multitasking, partly explain feeling exhausted at the end of day while thinking, "I got absolutely nothing done today."

Most of us need to work to relearn how to have singular focus. Think about not just doing one task at a time, but one type of task at a time. For example, devote fifteen to thirty minutes to email early in the workday, then ignore it for a while. Group administrative tasks for another concentrated block of work, then perhaps switch to more creative work. Take short breaks of physical activity between types of tasks. And, of course, shut out sources of distraction, such as pinging message notifications and "just a quick look" dives into social media sites.

You can further cultivate this ability to focus in non-work settings. When you're in line at the grocery store or waiting for a bus or standing outside a restaurant while your friend parks, resist the urge to look at your phone. Become accustomed to not having to be stimulated at all times. Just be present, and remind yourself it's good to give your brain a break.

#86: Value In-Person over Online Interactions

I have Facebook, Twitter, Instagram, Medium, and LinkedIn accounts; maintain a personal website; and regularly use collaborative project-management online tools for work. I've texted my wife when she's been elsewhere in the house. And I've been told I'm a great email correspondent.

So at least hear me out when I argue for prioritizing an in-person over online social life.

We'll see elsewhere in this chapter that enjoyable and health-boosting hormones are released in some common social situations, such as laughing, singing, and volunteering. We'll also see the

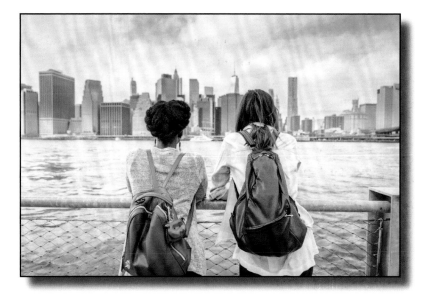

psychological benefits of the physical act of touch, and that feelings of isolation are associated with depression. These findings probably make intuitive sense to you on a subjective level—overall, it's likely you feel better after spending time in the physical presence of the people you really care about.

Contrast that with the findings of a now-famous study on Facebook users. For two weeks, researchers checked in five times a day and asked the subjects, "How do you feel right now?" They also asked about the subjects' amount of direct social interaction and Facebook use since the researchers last contacted them. The researchers had the subjects fill out a questionnaire about how satisfied they were with their lives before and after the two-week study.

The researchers found that the more people used Facebook, the worse they subsequently felt. In addition, the more the subjects used Facebook, the more their satisfaction with their lives declined over time. These findings did not happen in regard to the subjects' direct social interactions.

Consider these findings the mental health analogue of an idea from earlier chapters—modern conveniences can do more harm than good. Use online social interactions to complement, not replace, the more meaningful bonds built by personal presence.

#87: Challenge Your Brain

"My mind rebels at stagnation," Sherlock Holmes says in an early story. You could do worse than emulating one of the smartest fictional characters ever created. (Well, except for the cocaine and tobacco habits.)

Earlier in this chapter, we saw how regular aerobic exercise helps your neurons, the cells in the brain that transmit information to other cells. Synapses are the means by which they do that transmitting. When these connectors between neurons degenerate, your cognitive abilities decline. One key way to prevent that degradation is to regularly challenge your brain in specific ways; doing so strengthens existing connections and can spur new ones to be formed.

What kind of challenges encourage strong synapses? The word "challenge" is key—avoid routine. Of course, meeting daily responsibilities requires and even rewards some routine; you can't show up at work every morning and start from scratch in performing regular duties. But where possible, shake things up. Take up new hobbies that require learning new skills. Learn another language. Start a new activity that challenges your motor skills, or how well you can get your brain to make your body perform a desired movement. (An extreme example is juggling.) Take a class in a topic you avoided in earlier schooling. Take music lessons. Learn a craft. Recreate what was a common experience when you were growing up, that of regularly being taken out of your mental comfort zone.

These suggestions are not only for older adults. Indeed, some research suggests that starting new mental games late in life might not help much if cognitive decline has already started; taking up crossword puzzles then will mostly make you better only at doing crosswords. (Not that there's anything wrong with that, says the devotee of weekend *New York Times* puzzles.) As with physical exercise and other good habits, a lifetime approach might help prevent significant decline from starting.

#88: Take Up Knitting

No, this recommendation to knit or quilt or crochet hasn't errantly found its way into the mental health chapter. There are two key ways that these crafts can benefit your brain.

First, regardless of age, knitting has been shown to reduce stress, according to the Craft Yarn Council. In its surveys of knitters, the council has repeatedly found that practitioners list stress relief as one of their main reasons for knitting. The quiet concentration and gentle rhythmic movement involved in knitting can lower blood pressure and levels of the stress hormone cortisol similar to what occurs during meditation or yoga. The necessity of being present in the moment when knitting has been valued among people with depression and anxiety as a way to escape negative thought cycles.

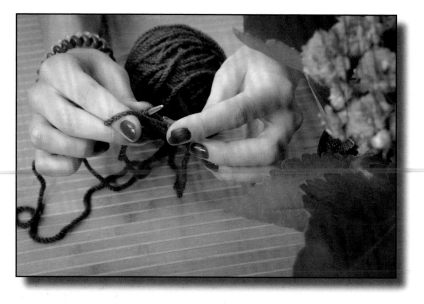

Second, for older people, knitting presents a neural challenge to the brain that fights cognitive decline. A Mayo Clinic study of people in their seventies and eighties found that those who did knitting and other crafts were less likely to incur cognitive impairment and memory loss. People in the study who did only non-tactile mental activities, such as reading, suffered greater declines.

#89: Practice Mindfulness Meditation

Research increasingly shows the mental-health benefits of one of the most popular forms of meditation, mindfulness. This practice doesn't mean burning incense and saying "Om." Researchers call it "training in present-focused awareness." It involves focusing your attention on the present rather than the past or future.

If you've tried mindfulness meditation, you know that clearing your mind to focus only on the present is difficult. Random thoughts will regularly pop up. Past regrets and future worries can appear out of nowhere. You might find yourself watching yourself tell yourself you're not supposed to be having those thoughts. Sitting quietly and being present is a great contrast to how we operate during much of modern daily life.

And that's why it's so good for you. One large-scale review of research found that mindfulness meditation helps to reduce anxiety, depression, and general feelings of stress. Other studies have shown benefits for those with insomnia and other sleep problems. All of these conditions are marked by negative thoughts that can seem to get stuck on automatic replay. Mindfulness meditation can help to break that cycle of thinking. Even if you're not clinically anxious or

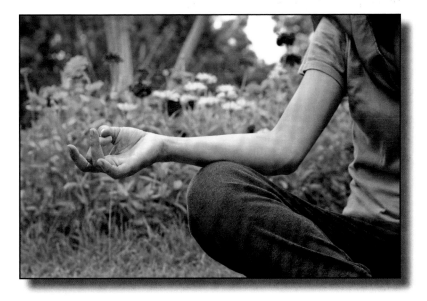

depressed, there's great relief in clearing a mind that's been racing all day, flitting from one microtask and deadline to another while worrying how you're going to get it all done. Over time, you'll be able to produce that state of mind in stressful situations as a way of calming and refocusing yourself.

To practice mindfulness meditation, find a comfortable place to sit with good posture in a quiet room. Focus on your inhalations and exhalations as you slowly belly breathe (see item #9). Your goal is to be free of goals, to simply be present as your mind gets a chance to unwind. If a stray thought about an unpleasant occurrence yesterday or an appointment tomorrow enters your mind, focus again on your breath and come back to the present. Sit like this for as long as feels comfortable. Setting a timer feels contrary to the spirit of the exercise, but if you can practice mindfulness meditation for ten to fifteen minutes most days, you'll see significant benefits.

#90: Take a Walk in Nature

A walk anywhere is good for your physical health. But for the most short-term mental benefits, research suggests strolling in nature is the way to go. According to research, our brains enter a more meditative state when we move from a typical city setting to a public green space.

In a study published a few years ago, researchers had people walk through Edinburgh, Scotland, while wearing a device that monitored their brain waves. The walkers started in a shopping district that has nineteenth-century buildings and light traffic. From there, they walked to a park. After a stroll there, they ended by walking through a busy commercial district that has lots of traffic and noise.

The walkers' brain activity varied greatly during their relatively brief tour (about twenty-five minutes total) of the three urban environments. In moving from the shopping district to the park, brain activity associated with frustration, engagement, and long-term arousal fell, while activity associated with meditation rose.

That changed when the walkers left the park and moved through the busy, loud commercial district. In that latter setting, one type of brain activity—"engagement or alertness with directed attention," the researchers called it—dominated. The walkers, in nonscientific terms, were on edge, just minutes after their brains showed signs of greater calm and inner focus.

Note that the walkers weren't deep in remote woods. They were in a small public green space that provided an oasis from

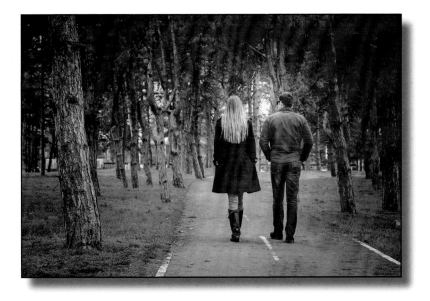

urban hustle and bustle. Such places abound. If you don't have easy access to one, it's worth the time and effort on nonworkdays to get yourself to a natural setting for a walk. Your brain will thank you.

#91: Time Your Caffeine Intake

A good cup of coffee or tea can improve your mood at just about any time of day. If you're happy with your caffeine routine and if it doesn't interfere with your sleep, there's no reason to change it. You can, however, make the most of caffeine's cognitive benefits by timing your enjoyment.

Elsewhere in this book, we've seen where elevated levels of the stress hormone cortisol can harm your health. Note the word "elevated"—cortisol-release cycles are a natural part of your circadian rhythm, helping you to feel more alert in the morning and more ready for sleep in the evening. In most people, cortisol levels rise between early and mid morning, taper off until early afternoon, have another, smaller rise, dip again, have a final rise in late afternoon, and decrease as evening falls.

Caffeine increases cortisol secretion. One school of thought says that you should avoid caffeine when your body is programmed to naturally secrete cortisol. The theory is that having caffeine at these times interferes with your circadian rhythms. In addition, the thinking goes, having caffeine at these times increases your tolerance and therefore lowers caffeine's effectiveness. What's better, according to this model, is to have caffeine when your body's cortisol levels are falling, in the late morning and midafternoon.

As someone who loves starting the day talking with my wife while we enjoy our coffee, I've chosen to treat the above thinking as an instance where logic tells me one thing and emotion another. For now, I'm sticking with my first-thing-in-the-morning coffee. But there appears to be sound science here that's worth investigating if you're not as wed to the morning ritual.

Like many people, I drink more than one cup of coffee a day. And like many people, I've instinctively gravitated toward having my second (and, yes, sometimes third) cup in synch with the cortisol-release cycle described above. That's because caffeine aids certain types of mental tasks, some of which our work compels us to do regardless of our falling cortisol levels.

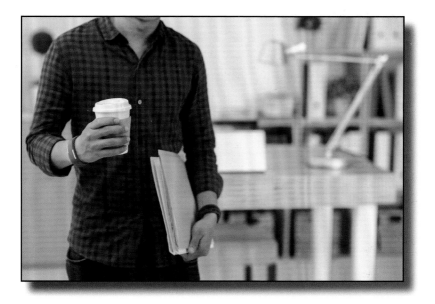

For starters, caffeine increases alertness and attention. No duh, right? What's helpful here is knowing that it can take twenty to forty-five minutes for caffeine to be fully absorbed. So if you know you'll have a task requiring heightened alertness, don't wait until you feel like you're lagging. Time your caffeine so that when it kicks in coincides with when you need to be vigilant.

The same thinking applies to the speed with which you work. Here, things are a little more nuanced. Caffeine boosts productivity on relatively straightforward mental-processing tasks. It will help you plow through a pile of invoices, for example, but is unlikely to assist when you're doing more abstract or creative thinking.

Caffeine probably also helps with working memory, such as recalling a list of names or dates. This appears to especially be the case in what one researcher called "suboptimal alertness conditions," or what most people call feeling tired. The takeaway: time your caffeine intake to coincide with when you'll be doing the sorts of mental work it aids, especially if you'll be doing those tasks when your cortisol levels are naturally waning.

You don't need to down a double espresso to get these benefits. One study found increased performance on mental-processing tests after subjects had as little 12.5 milligrams of caffeine. By way of comparison, an eight-ounce cup of green tea, considered one of the "weakest" teas, contains between 25 and 70 milligrams of caffeine, depending in part on brewing time. This finding supports many people's habit of drinking tea in the afternoon for a milder version of the caffeine buzz they enjoyed via coffee in the morning. It's a good strategy if you need help being alert at work but don't want to risk compromising your sleep.

#92: Consider Light Therapy in the Winter

Seasonal affective disorder is a form of depression that predictably occurs at one time of the year but doesn't affect the person the rest of the year. It can occur in people who are otherwise mostly free of depressive symptoms in other seasons or on top of chronic depressive symptoms. Symptoms include sleep disruptions, low energy, irritability, problems with social interactions, and weight gain.

The most common time to experience seasonal affective disorder, or SAD, is the winter. It's thought that one cause is the seasonal change in the amount and type of sunlight. This theory is

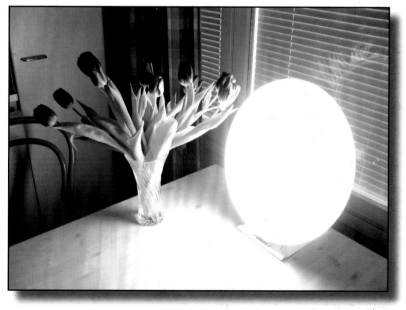

Image via Creative Commons

supported by the fact that SAD is much more prevalent in places like Alaska and Finland than Florida.

A partial solution is light therapy, which consists of sitting by a light box that mimics outdoor light. Regular exposure is believed to alter brain chemistry sufficiently to ease some of the symptoms of SAD. Light therapy is thought to be most effective if done soon after you wake, for twenty to thirty minutes. The box should be set up sixteen to twenty-four inches from you so that you're exposed to the light but not looking at it. It's easy to integrate light therapy into a typical morning routine, such as setting it where you have morning coffee and/or check your phone or laptop.

A good light-therapy box or lamp will emit at least 10,000 lux of light, with little to none of that being ultraviolet light. These can be found for about $100.

Don't wait for SAD to strike before starting light therapy. Daylight hours begin to diminish rapidly in October in the Northern Hemisphere. That's a good time to establish a light-therapy routine in the hope of lessening the severity of symptoms come December and the shortest days of the year.

If you're affected by SAD, you can also lessen its hold on you by taking proactive steps such as regular exercise, getting outside during the limited daylight hours, and engaging in social activities, even if it takes an effort to place yourself in these situations.

#93: Volunteer

Help yourself by helping others. Research has found that there's merit to this seemingly paradoxical idea.

The good feeling you get from selfless acts stems from dopamine, a neurotransmitter in your brain that's released during pleasurable behavior. The activities that lead to dopamine release are generally those your body wants to reward you for doing, because they're somehow in your body's interest for you to repeat. So the same chemical associated with things like sex, food, and exercise is released during altruistic activities. It's believed this occurs because humans evolved as social animals; those whose bodies rewarded cooperative behavior were more likely to reproduce and pass on their genes.

In addition, nearly all volunteering entails social interaction and collaborative effort, which help to reduce the feelings of isolation and loneliness associated with depression.

In one intriguing study, women over the age of sixty-five who volunteered remained consistent or even improved on tests of brain executive function, which include cognitive processes like working memory and the ability to pay attention. A control group of age-matched women saw no such gains.

As with so many topics we've looked at in this book, volunteering simultaneously aids the brain and body. One study found that people over the age of fifty who volunteered regularly were less likely to develop high blood pressure than nonvolunteers. In a different study, people over the age of sixty-five who volunteered regularly had a significantly lower risk of dying during the study period than those who didn't volunteer. Of course, it's possible that healthier people are better able to volunteer. But there's enough evidence about the health benefits of volunteering to suggest this needn't be an unresolvable chicken-or-egg question.

#94: Experience Touch

The health benefits of being touched are a great example of the porous boundary between physical phenomena and mental state.

Research on hugging has found that a warm embrace from a loved one releases oxytocin, a hormone that acts as a neurotransmitter in the brain. Elevated oxytocin levels are associated with the glow that accompanies bonding, be it romantic, parental, or personal. Oxytocin also strengthens the immune system, suggesting that regular meaningful touch can make you less susceptible to colds and other illnesses.

At the same time, touch has been found to lower stress. Being touched can decrease levels of cortisol, the fight-or-flight hormone

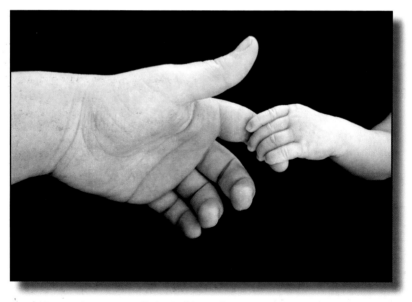

Image via Creative Commons

that elevates blood pressure. And get this: in one fascinating study, researchers administered functional MRIs on women who were told they might get a slight electrical shock. While anticipating the potential shock, the women's brains showed increased activity associated with anxiety. But that brain activity while waiting for something bad to happen quieted when they held hands, either with a researcher or their husbands. (The husbands reading this will be happy to hear the women experienced greater stress relief in the latter situation.)

These benefits of touch occur not just with loved ones. Part of the stress relief most people feel from a massage is thought to be from the release of oxytocin and lowered cortisol levels and blood pressure. The latest occupation to benefit from the human need for touch? Professional snugglers, who provide platonic spooning and other nonsexual forms of touch that can be hard to find in an age of digital distraction and virtual friendships.

#95: Laugh

When someone says, "I could use a good laugh," they're not just mouthing a cliché. They're intuitively recognizing the stress relief and improved mood laughter can provide.

Laughter spurs the release of certain neuropeptides, which are small proteins that facilitate communication between neurons, either via the blood to work on receptors in the body or in the brain to activate receptors there. The upshot is an uptick in brain and/or bodily activity that is health-enhancing.

Among the things that happen when you laugh are an initial arousal but then calming of your stress-response system, increased oxygenation of organs and other tissues, release of feel-good endorphins, and muscle relaxation (once you get over the hysterical, holding-your-sides phase).

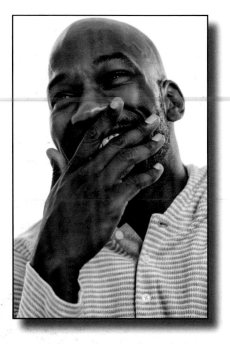

The regular occurrence of these good processes can mean a stronger immune system and less chronic pain, as the body frequently produces natural painkillers.

Try to regularly place yourself in laugh-inducing situations. That can be the presence of funny friends, YouTube clips of a favored comedian, a good comedy at the theater, even books. Laughter is a social phenomenon—you're likely to laugh harder at something when others are present. If you've ever been in a room when a good stand-up comic is nailing it, you know the special feeling that comes from group laughter.

Laughter might not always be the best medicine, but it's one that's worth taking daily.

#96: Sing

Looking for an oxytocin release but can't find someone to reach out and touch? Try belting out a few of your favorite songs.

That's just one of the mental benefits of singing. It's also been found to release endorphins, the body's natural opiates responsible for the famous "runner's high."

Perhaps because there was an evolutionary advantage to group cohesion, the mental benefits of singing seem to be especially strong when you're part of a choir. That's consistent with the release of oxytocin; and, as we saw in item #94, it's associated with bonding and trust. Research on group singing has found that just one hour of practice lowers participants' anxiety levels. Longer-term studies have found reductions in depressive symptoms and improvements in overall quality-of-life assessments from consistent choir membership.

Research suggests the always-welcome endorphin release isn't unique to singing. In separate studies on singers, drummers, and dancers, an Oxford University researcher found greater pain

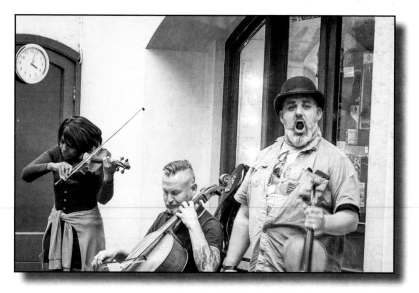

Image via Creative Commons

tolerance after all these forms of musical performance and attributed the finding to endorphin release. No wonder Ringo Starr is so happy and healthy.

#97: Name Your Emotions

One way to improve your mental state when you feel bad is to think about the matter deeply enough to say more than, "I feel bad."

The psychologist Lisa Feldman Barrett calls naming negative emotions with precision "emotional granularity." For example, instead of "I feel bad," you might say, "I'm depressed," or, "I'm lonely," or, "I'm anxious."

The value in these more precise statements is that they better allow you to address the negative emotion. If you're depressed, you might examine whether things are as hopeless as they appear. If you're lonely, you might look at the quality of your social network. If you're anxious, you might identify causes of anxiety and plan how to deal with them.

According to Feldman Barrett, people who are better at emotional granularity are less likely to engage in self-defeating behaviors such as drinking too much or lashing out at others. After all, if you merely say, "I'm miserable," drinking yourself to sleep might seem like a good solution. But if you say, "I'm lonely," then you're more likely to realize that getting drunk is going to do nothing to better your situation.

Over time, more precisely naming negative emotions should help you realize the areas in your life most in need of improvement.

If most of your statements have to do with despondency, then your focus will be different than if you most often speak of anxiety.

#98: Ask for Help When You Need It

Here's the flip side of volunteering. We all need help sometimes. Asking for it accomplishes important things.

First, it clearly identifies the problem. Depending on the issue, giving name to it could be the initial step in improving a lifelong struggle. Being as specific as possible will allow a better plan of attack and give useful guidance to those whose help you seek.

Second, asking for help makes you be honest with yourself. You've identified a situation that is beyond your power to fix at the moment. Reflecting on how you got in the situation can help you to avoid it in the future.

Third, realizing the situation is beyond your power to fix at the moment can be liberating. You don't expect others to be self-contained automatons, so why put that pressure on yourself?

Similarly, asking for help should lower feelings of isolation and hopelessness. Your mood should improve as you realize you're not alone and that you've started a process to improve things. Your request for help will almost certainly be granted by those close to you, strengthening your bond and lessening the chance that you'll feel as isolated in the future.

A final point: there's no shame in seeking help from a professional such as a counselor or psychiatrist. Your health is too important to sacrifice to the belief that doing so is a sign of weakness.

#99: Write a Thank You Letter

Researchers have found a surprising number of psychological and physical benefits from gratitude, or acknowledging what's good in your life. People who regularly express gratitude have been found to be happier, more resilient in the face of adversity, in better health, and better sleepers.

Some of this research has been conducted on people who keep gratitude journals, in which they write about people, things,

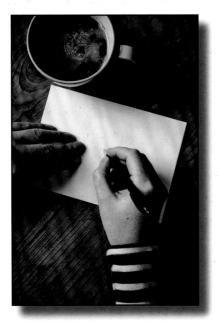

occasions, etc., that they're grateful for. That's a good practice if you need to be reminded that, actually, yours probably isn't the most miserable existence in human history.

But why not let others know? After all, inherent in gratitude is a recognition that many of the things you're thankful for are external. In many cases, that's something that someone else has done for you. Realizing this is part of why gratitude is good for mental health, because it reduces feelings of isolation and even hopelessness.

Once you've identified people who have made your world a better place, take five minutes and send them a text, an email, or, best yet, a handwritten note. Think of what joy you would get receiving such a note, and how, with little effort, you could provide that joy to someone who helped you. The person may well have forgotten doing what you're thanking them for, but they will long remember your act of gratitude. You'll benefit as well: in one study, people who delivered a thank-you letter saw their happiness increase significantly, and it stayed elevated for a month.

#100: Don't Be a Martyr

At the beginning of this book, I suggested applying the concept of choice architecture to your health endeavors. That was a practical recommendation—make it easy to implement good health habits. I'll conclude by making a parallel psychological recommendation— make it easy to think the right way about good health habits.

Doing so is matter of framing how you think about your health practices. When you institute changes, it's natural to think in terms of sacrifice, of getting yourself to do something you don't want to do: "I'm giving up food X because I was told it's bad for me" or "I have to get up and exercise tomorrow before work." This martyrly mindset is not a fun one to live by (or be around), because it makes tending to your health feel like a burden and like you're constantly denying yourself. It can also make you feel like you're not really in control of your life.

An alternative way to think about the same practices is to consider them choices: "I'm choosing not to eat food X because it will not improve my health," or "I'm choosing to exercise before work tomorrow because it will improve my health and make the rest of my day better." This mindset reinforces that you're doing things for the sake of one of your most precious possessions, your health. It puts you in control. It's a way of saying to yourself and others, "Here's how I'm choosing to live, and my life is better for my doing so."

Make choices, not sacrifices. I hope that this book has given you several ideas about choices you can make today to improve your health and life. *À votre santé* !

Acknowledgments

Jay Cassell and Rob Wilson were helpful in getting this project going, and Stacey Cramp was supportive while I saw it to completion. I'm honored that Phil Wharton wrote the foreword and that Alex Hutchinson, Michael Joyner, and Bill Roberts were willing to read an in-process manuscript and comment positively on it.

About the Author

Scott Douglas is a contributing editor for *Runner's World*. He is the author or co-author of seven other books, including *The Little Red Book of Running* and the *New York Times* best seller *Meb for Mortals*. He has written on fitness and health for *The Atlantic*, *Slate*, the *Washington Post,* and others. Scott lives in South Portland, Maine, and tries his best to follow his own advice.

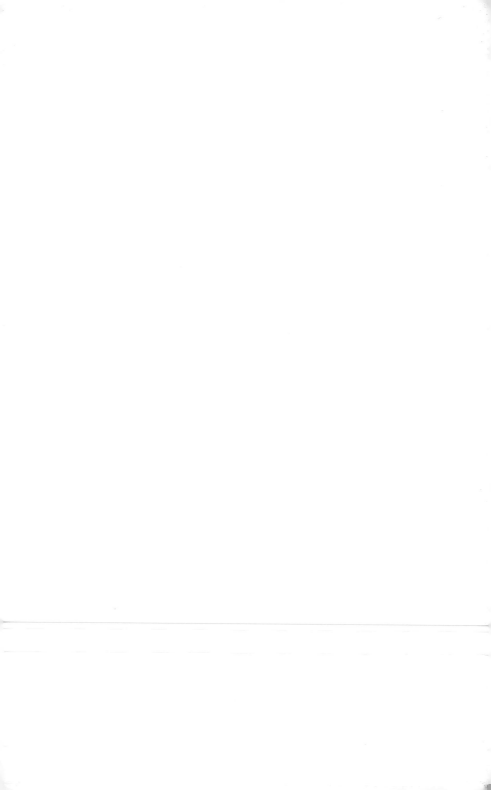